616.834
ROG

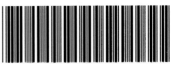

369 0290597

…rosis: Answers at your fi…

'Written by experts in the condition in a practical and accessible format,
ideal for anyone to get both an overview and the latest up-to-date
information required.

PHIL BAZLEY (who has MS), Chairman,
Greater Manchester Neurological Association

'. . . an extremely useful and comprehensive resource for the UK MS
community.'

The Multiple Sclerosis Society

'Authoritative and …………… a …uable resource for all those affected
by MS.'

…e Multiple Sclerosis Trust

'I thought I already knew everything there was to know about MS, but this
book has made me feel even more knowledgeable! I think it will be a very
useful book for anyone recently diagnosed with MS, and will continue to be
useful throughout their lives.'

LOUISE SHAW (who has MS), London

19.99

D1420132

Comments on the first edition

'My overall impression is of excellence and comprehensiveness. The thoroughness of the approach is much needed, as MS is so complex and individual.'

JAN HATCH, Former Director of Services, MS Society

'I found it easy to read and understand. My wife Pam could easily relate to much of the contents.'

ALLAN QUARTLEY, Somerset

'It is delightful to find a book that does not go into so much medical detail as to make it incomprehensible to the lay person, yet still covers the various options that an MS sufferer has available in the management of the illness. What I found most useful is that this is a book that you can give to your relatives and friends in order to ease their comprehension of the illness.'

EDITH J PASTERNAK-ALBERT

'I took early retirement when I was 44 years old and have learnt to take things in my stride. Every so often other things crop up and this book will be a fabulous reference for me.'

DELFINA WALKER

Multiple sclerosis

Answers at your fingertips

Dr David Rog BMedSci (Hons), BM, BS, MD, MRCP
Megan Burgess BSc (Hons), RGN, PG Dip, MSCN
Dr John Mottershead BM, BCh, BA (Oxon), FRCP
and **Dr Paul Talbot** MB, CHB, MD, FRCP

CLASS PUBLISHING · LONDON

The information presented in this book is accurate and current to the best of the authors' knowledge. The authors and publisher, however, make no guarantee as to, and assume no responsibility for, the correctness, sufficiency or completeness of such information or recommendation. The reader is advised to consult a doctor regarding all aspects of individual health care.

Printing history
First published 2000
Second edition 2010

The authors and publisher welcome feedback from the users of this book. Please contact the publisher.
Class Publishing, Barb House, Barb Mews, London W6 7PA, UK
Telephone: (020) 7371 2119
Fax: (020) 7371 2878 [International +4420]
Email: post@class.co.uk
Visit our website – www.class.co.uk

A CIP catalogue record for this book is available from the British Library

ISBN 978 1 85959 218 2

10 9 8 7 6 5 4 3 2 1

Designed and typeset by Martin Bristow

Cartoons by Jane Taylor

Illustrations by David Woodroffe

Edited by Richenda Milton-Daws

Printed and bound in Gateshead by Athenaeum Press

Contents

Foreword

by **Simon Gillespie**
Chief Executive, the MS Society

MS is a condition that is unique in its unpredictability and for the 50 people diagnosed every week this uncertainty will be difficult to live with.

It can cause one or more of a broad range of symptoms from chronic fatigue to nerve pain, loss of sight and mobility, depression, loss of memory, mood swings, incontinence, sexual dysfunction and spasticity.

No one can say what the future impact of the disease will be; MS affects everyone diagnosed differently. This uncertainty about the future and the unpredictability of the present, however, is the most disabling aspect of MS, and that is why accurate information is so important.

There is plenty of information out there but not all of it reliable, especially on the Internet – often the first place people go when they have questions about the condition. It is only reliable and comprehensive answers to the wide range of questions that people with MS have that will enable them to make informed decisions about their present and future.

Multiple sclerosis: Answers at your fingertips takes questions that have been asked by people affected by MS, and offers accessible, clear answers. Thus, it is an extremely useful reference book for the UK MS community.

The comprehensive content will be an invaluable resource to many people living with this unpredictable and fluctuating disease, enabling them to make choices for themselves.

Simon Gillespie

Foreword

by **Chris Jones**
Trustee and co-founder, the MS Trust

Multiple sclerosis is a condition known for its complexity, unpredictability and uncertainty.

It is most often diagnosed in people in their 20s and 30s at a time when life style, family, relationship and career decisions are being made. It is not a time when you expect to be given a diagnosis of a chronic and potentially disabling condition. That is for old people. Most of us are completely unprepared for such a life-changing event and the overwhelming need is to know more. What is happening to the body I thought I could rely on? Why me? What treatment is there? What can I do for myself? This book seeks to answer, in a clear and straightforward way, all these questions – and many more.

MS is beset by myths and the less responsible media constantly offer false hope. Well-meaning friends tell us about 'miracle cures' they spotted, usually on the Internet.

This is the value of reliable information: it enables those who are affected by MS, whether personally or through a family member or friend, to sift the hype and false claims and to find out what is right for them. Understanding the condition – and recognising its many uncertainties – are the tools needed to take control of their lives and make informed decisions.

Armed with this knowledge, I still have MS but MS doesn't have me.

Chris Jones

Acknowledgements

To all our patient with MS, your courage and good humour is an inspiration. Thank you for continuing to teach and inform us.

We are grateful to our colleagues at *Greater Manchester Neurosciences Centre, based at Salford Royal NHS Foundation Trust* – in particular the MS specialist nurses: Alison, Chris, Denise, Liz, Fran and Wendy. Their contributions and suggestions have been invaluable.

We would never have finished writing this book without the wonderful support of our partners and families. Special mention must be made of Jozef, Vera, Zoe, Jack and Isobel Rog, David and Becky Burgess, Naomi, Tom and Johnny Mottershead, and Anne, Hannah and Beth Talbot, all of whom have demonstrated admirable patience during the writing process. Thank you so much. And thanks too to Diane for her friendship.

**David Rog, Megan Burgess,
John Mottershead and Paul Talbot**

Introduction

Whether you are a person with MS, a person who is concerned they may have MS, or a relative, friend or carer of someone with MS, we wrote this book for you. Over the years, health professionals like us cannot help but get to know many people with MS, along with their families and friends. We are in the privileged position of hearing their hopes, aspirations and fears, and of sharing some of the good and bad times.

It is ten years since Professor Ian Robinson, Dr Stuart Neilson and Professor Frank Clifford Rose wrote the first edition of this book, and we are grateful to them for setting the benchmark. We hope that we have built upon their efforts, taking into account the many developments that have occurred in MS care, management and research over that time.

So, when Class Publishing approached us to update the previous edition of *Multiple Sclerosis: Answers at your fingertips*, we were delighted to accept. We believe that, although there are now a number of excellent resources for people with MS, none answer the broad range of practical questions that we are commonly asked, in such an effective format. We hope that you will find thorough and honest answers to many of the questions that you, or someone you love, may have.

Our author team is made up of three consultant neurologists and a nurse consultant, all of whom specialise in MS and have long-term practical experience. We work closely with MS specialist nurses, who we thank for their suggestions and input to this book. We also thank the many people with MS, and their relatives, who contributed questions.

In Manchester we run regular courses for people newly diagnosed with MS and their loved ones, and a number of the new questions in this edition arose directly from people who attended these sessions. In this way we hope that this book answers the questions to which you want answers.

WHERE IS OUR EVIDENCE?

This is not a textbook. You won't find references to specific studies, for example, but in the Appendices there are a whole host of resources that you may find helpful if you want to find further information. The opinions expressed are our own, and where possible are formed by the results of clinical trials but sometimes the formal evidence is lacking and in these cases it is based upon our experience of helping people with MS manage their illness. Some opinions will not necessarily be shared by all other practitioners. However, for much of the clinical and statistical information, we have drawn upon the classic medical textbook in the field, *McAlpine's Multiple Sclerosis* by Alistair Compston, Ian McDonald, John Noseworthy and others. The fourth (and current) edition was published in 2006 by Churchill Livingstone.

We have also made use of a number of learned articles, several of which deserve special mention. Professor Compston, Dr Coles and their team, in a number of published articles outlining their pioneering work with the drug Campath 1H (Alemtuzumab) have effectively demonstrated a 'two-stage model' of MS. Dr Mike Boggild has published a case series of his experience relating to drug treatment of MS with mitoxantrone. Alvaro Alonso and colleagues published an article on the incidence of MS in the UK in the *Journal of Neurology* in 2007, and we have drawn upon their findings too.

We have also learned a great deal from people like you, and we welcome your feedback on this edition.

HOW YOU MIGHT USE THIS BOOK

This book is not designed to be read from cover to cover (although we have all done so several times and there is some repetition if you do choose to). Although there are symptoms in MS which are common to a number of people, everyone's illness and experience is unique to them, as is the way they choose to manage their MS.

The fact that you are reading this suggests that you do wish to know more. Class Publishing designed the *Answers at your Fingertips* series to have a common layout, as a series of questions and answers arranged in chapters. There is a glossary of terms at the back of the book and words explained it are in *italics* the first time they appear in the body of the book. There are also lists of useful addresses, further reading and other resources, and some key medical information in the Appendices.

Some of you will choose to read the whole of this book in one go, others will purposefully read a small section that you think will be relevant to you at a particular point in your illness. There may be long periods when you put it back on the shelf to gather dust, and hope that you won't need it. Others will pick it up occasionally, dip in and check whether a new symptom, treatment, or drug you have heard about in the media or from other people is worth considering in more detail. Some of you, as carers and loved ones, will read this to get some insight into what having MS means.

We hope that you find the book useful in whichever way you choose to use it. If you feel there are any glaring omissions or new questions that you would like the answers to, please contact Class Publishing at the address on the back cover or this book or on info@class.co.uk. We will try to include your suggestions in any revisions.

Answers to the questions you feel you cannot ask!

You may be uncomfortable about asking certain types of questions, for example regarding the unusual and bizarre qualities of nerve pain ('Am I imagining it?') or about the impact of MS on your sex life, whether it is you or your partner who has MS. You may feel that these issues affect only you or your loved one but, as you will see, this is unlikely to be the case. In our experience, many of your queries and concerns are actually very similar. We hope that you will get at least an outline of why we think particular symptoms occur, or about some of the treatments that are available to you or, conversely, why some treatments may not be suitable for you.

Remember to use your local MS Team

However successful we may or may not have been in answering your questions, this book is no substitute for engaging with *your* neurologist, ms nurse, GP and other members of the team. But beware – it may arm you with even more questions! We hope this book will help you get the most out of your contacts with *your* MS team. MS is a lifelong illness and a good relationship with your team is crucial to help you manage your illness effectively.

Are we always right?

We have generally erred on the side of caution where evidence is lacking in proving the effects of potential treatments, and have tried to give a balanced view. Members of your team may feel we are too cautious or perhaps not cautious enough and may disagree with our views. This is not unusual in medicine and does not necessarily imply that either of us is right! Any disagreements should at least prompt a discussion and an agreed approach.

There are commonly reports in the media of new treatments and potential 'cures' for MS. But, as we say in the book, it is important to look beyond the headline and carefully consider whether the substance of the article backs up the claim. 'Show me the evidence' is always a good approach to take.

Thank you!

Finally, although we have written this book for you, *we* have learned from our previous and existing patients and their families and from patients who have participated in clinical studies. Thank you to them for their selflessness and good humour. Their courage in living and dealing with this challenging illness is truly humbling.

David Rog, Megan Burgess, John Mottershead and Paul Talbot

1 | What is multiple sclerosis (MS)?

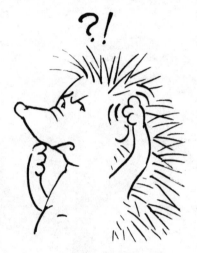

This chapter begins to explain our current understanding of what is happening in multiple sclerosis (MS). We then consider the *epidemiology* of the condition (which people are more likely to develop MS, whether where they live makes a difference, and whether the chance of developing MS is increasing). The rest of this book is concerned with the symptoms and other consequences of having MS and how they are best managed.

What is multiple sclerosis (MS)?

Multiple sclerosis (MS) is a disorder which involves the central nervous system, that is the brain and spinal cord. Currently MS is an incurable condition and therefore is lifelong once it develops. Certain areas of the brain such as the optic (eye) nerves, are more commonly affected than others (see Figure 1.1).

In MS, areas of inflammation or swelling develop which can be demonstrated as white dots on MRI scans. These abnormal areas are

A midline view of the brain

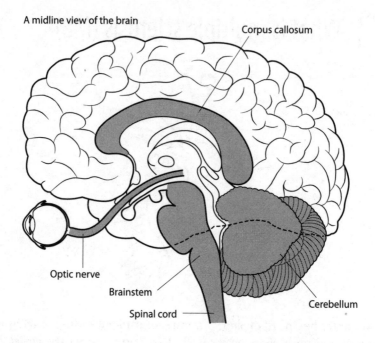

Figure 1.1 Areas of the brain commonly affected by MS

referred to as *plaques* and when they cause major symptoms they are described as a *relapse*. Relapses cause short-term disability. The extent of recovery depends upon the success of the body's repair systems.

Currently, we believe that MS is a two-stage illness: inflammation and relapses predominate early on in the illness, while the death of nerve cells (a process called neurodegeneration) is thought to be responsible for long term and progressive disability. Exactly when or whether long-term nerve cell loss is 'programmed', and whether it is triggered by inflammation or occurs independently of it, are some of the fundamental unanswered questions about MS. The treatments that are available at present reduce inflammation and relapses. However, no treatments have been shown, beyond question, to reduce substantially the progression of long-term disability.

So if MS is a disorder of the nervous system, what actually happens to the nerves?

The purpose of the nervous system is to convey messages, which travel along nerves as small electric impulses (see Figure 1.2). You can think of nerve cells as electrical wires. Messages, in the form of electrical currents, are passed from the brain along the nerves to the muscles – for example, in the arms and legs – enabling us to move. Sensations travel from the periphery to the brain, and thus allow us to feel. In order to increase the speed and reliability with which these electrical messages are carried (conducted) along the nerves, they are lagged or insulated by a substance called myelin, just as copper wires are insulated by a plastic coating. As a result, there is normally no change in the size of the electrical signal from one end of the nerve to the other.

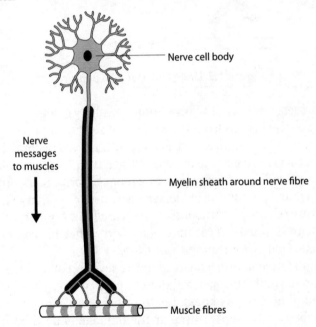

Figure 1.2 A neuron

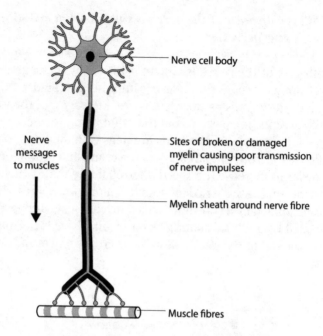

Figure 1.3 Demyelination of a neuron

MS causes areas of inflammation (swelling), which leads to stripping of the myelin from the surface of nerves, a process called demyelination (see Figure 1.3). As a result, nerves become far less reliable at carrying electrical messages along their length. Sometimes the messages will get through but in a reduced form. Sometimes the messages may be temporarily delayed because of a change in body temperature (*Uhthoff's phenomenon*, see below). And sometimes these frayed, demyelinated nerves may react with other nerves, causing spontaneous pains, for example (see Chapter 12).

Inflammation can also lead to complete severing of a nerve. If this occurs, no normal messages will then be carried along it. This could lead to numbness or weakness. Death of nerve cells may also result from the body's attempts to repair the damage caused by inflammation. Sometimes, damaged nerve cells are replaced by non-nerve

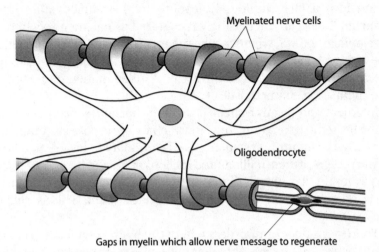

Myelinated nerve cells

Oligodendrocyte

Gaps in myelin which allow nerve message to regenerate

Figure 1.4 An oligodendrocyte

cells called glial cells, with harmful results. Glial cells support nerve cells in a framework but also have many other functions, including the production of myelin by a particular type of glial cell called an oligodendrocyte (see Figure 1.4). The replacement of nerve cells by glial cells is called gliosis and gives rise to the scarring (*multiple scleroses*) from where multiple *sclerosis* gets its name.

What causes MS? I have heard it is something to do with the immune system – is this correct?

The cause of MS remains unknown, but the immune system plays a central role in its development. The human immune system has two major groups of cells that help fight infection. The first are *T-cells* (also known as *T-lymphocytes*) which take foreign substances into them, before repackaging components of these on their surface to influence the actions of other cells. The second are *B-cells* (also known as *B-lymphocytes*) which produce *antibodies* – proteins of a complementary shape to foreign substances which attach to them like a key fitting into a lock, ultimately leading to their inactivation and removal. B-cells are increasingly recognised as having a role in the development of MS, whether it be the presence of oligoclonal bands (see Figure 4.3 in Chapter 4 on Diagnosis of MS) and antibodies in the cerebrospinal fluid, or in the areas of inflammation in the brain and spinal cord characteristic of MS.

In order to protect us from all potentially harmful substances such as the bacteria, viruses and fungi to which we are exposed throughout our lives, the immune system needs the flexibility to be able to adapt to and recognise these millions and millions of foreign items. The price we pay for this flexibility is that sometimes the immune cells recognise parts of our bodies as 'foreign' and attack them. This is called *autoreactivity*.

There a number of disorders where the body's own cells become autoreactive. In the case of rheumatoid arthritis, the body's own cells react against the joints. In MS, the autoreactive T-cells gain the ability to get from the bloodstream, across the blood brain barrier, and into the brain and spinal cord, where they trigger a series of events that result in the stripping of the lagging (myelin) around nerve cells (see Figure 1.3, above). This is called *demyelination*. Death of nerve cells can also occur causing permanent disability.

Whether or not inflammation accounts for all subsequent nerve cell death is one of the fundamental, and as yet unanswered, questions in MS. Current treatments have varying effects on inflammation but, at present, re-growth of nerve cells in the brain and spinal cord is impossible and protection of existing nerve cells is not proven.

Can you explain a bit more about why this myelin is important?

Myelin is produced by a type of glial cell called an oligodendrocyte. Each oligodendrocyte has many processes or legs which each end in a 'foot' of myelin and can help to insulate up to forty nerve cells in its surrounding area.

There are small gaps in the myelin, which allow the electrical message to continue to regenerate itself as it passes along the nerve.

Therefore, the message that is sent from one of end of the nerve is received both quickly and without distortion at the other end of the nerve.

During an acute attack when T-cells trigger demyelination, the nerve may not carry the electrical messages very well. This leads to weakness or altered sensation, for example. If the message is blocked and doesn't reach its target at all, this can lead to paralysis or numbness. The inflammation during an attack leads to a plaque or *lesion* which can sometimes be demonstrated on an MRI scan. The scarring, or *sclerosis*, that is left behind to varying degrees after a demyelinating plaque gives multiple sclerosis its name.

When the myelin is stripped away from nerves in MS, the oligodendrocytes tend to increase in number and try to repair the damage to the myelin by making a new supply. The repair process is never as good as the original: the myelin sheaths are typically thinner and shorter than before (see Figure 1.4), which means that electrical messages cannot be carried as efficiently. There are several possible consequences, described below.

The repair process may be good enough for you not to experience a symptom while you are at rest. However, your nerve is no longer properly insulated, and is therefore more prone to external influences such as changes in temperature. *Uhthoff's phenomenon* describes symptoms which worsen with increasing temperature, leading to a temporary reduction in the conduction of messages along an already damaged nerve. An example is blurring or loss of vision which may be brought about by exercise, a hot bath or shower, or even a hot drink in someone with a previously damaged eye (optic) nerve. As the body temperature returns to normal, so too does the speed of conduction of electrical impulses and vision. Incidentally, there is no additional damage to the nerve because of short-lived changes in body temperature.

The repair process may not be good enough and the conduction speed along the nerve remains lower than normal. You may therefore have permanent symptoms such as weakness, reduced vision or sensation.

The inflammation may be so bad as to cut or sever the nerve completely. This part of the nerve will now stop functioning and the whole nerve may die. Sometimes the nerve will remain alive and the stump at the level of the damage will become irritable and carry messages spontaneously or become activated at lower levels than is normal. It may also short circuit adjacent nerves. This can lead to a 'double whammy' situation: because the nerve is badly damaged, it does not carry normal impulses, but it is irritable and carries inappropriate impulses sometimes without being stimulated. This could result in a limb which is weak and stiff, going into spasm or spontaneously feeling burning, aching or sharp pain in an area of skin which otherwise feels numb (see Chapter 13 for more about pain, spasm and altered sensations). Alternatively, the pressure of bedsheets or the texture of certain types of material against the skin can feel painful as nerves which normally carry these sensations are inappropriately activated.

I heard my doctor talking about the 'blood-brain barrier'. What is that and what does it have to do with MS?

The *blood-brain barrier* (BBB) is formed by the interaction of the inner lining cells of blood vessels within the brain (*endothelium*), the nerve cells themselves and non-nerve supporting (*glial*) cells. Its roles include protecting the brain from substances within the bloodstream, which it does by restricting their physical passage into the brain and by processing substances within the blood before they reach the brain. The BBB also regulates the supply of sugar and other nutrients needed by the brain for it to function properly.

The BBB's relevance in MS is that, under normal circumstances, it closely regulates and restricts the passage of cells of the immune system from the blood to the brain. The passage of cells seems to be a crucial step in the development of MS, as the T-cells in MS react against parts of the brain itself. Some treatments are either specifically designed to reduce this passage of cells (e.g. *natalizumab*), or achieve this as one of their effects (*beta-inteferons* and *corticosteroids*).

HOW MANY PEOPLE GET MS, AND WHO ARE THEY?

How many people have MS?

At any time, approximately one out of every thousand people in the UK has MS. New cases of MS are diagnosed in around one in 15,000 people in the UK every year. The estimated lifetime risk of a man in the UK developing MS is one in 500 and for a woman one in 200. The lifetime risk is more than the one in a thousand mentioned earlier. This is largely because MS tends to affect adults, with the many children in the population unlikely to be at risk of MS. One way to understand this is to imagine a condition that affects everyone in a population, but that starts only at the age of 40. The lifetime risk of this condition would be close to 100 per cent. At any time, however, only about 50 per cent of the population would be affected, with those under the age of 40 being free of that condition. This is a major reason why the lifetime risk of MS is higher than the rate in the population at any one time.

Who usually gets MS?

MS is often considered to be a disease of young adults because it is usually diagnosed in people in their 20s to 40s. It is uncommon for it to start in childhood, and it is unlikely to develop later on in life. However, a particular form of MS, primary progressive MS, often presents at a later age with people developing symptoms in their 40s or 50s.

Although women are approximately twice as likely as men to get relapsing-remitting MS, roughly equal numbers of men and women get the less common primary progressive form of the condition. It appears that MS is much more common in white European (Caucasian) people than those of black African, Asian, Chinese or Japanese descent.

Studies have shown that the children, brothers, sisters and

non-identical twins of someone with MS (first-degree relatives) are at greater risk of getting MS than an unrelated person in the general population. This is probably because blood relatives share some of the genes that increase the likelihood of developing the condition. In fact, the lifetime risk for these particular first-degree relatives is around 1 in 30 (3 per cent) compared to 1 in 500 (0.2 per cent) in the general population. In comparison, nephews and nieces (second-degree relatives) and half-siblings share a lifetime risk between that of first-degree relatives and the general population – 1 in 100 (1 per cent). When considering these facts it is very important to appreciate that, even though some blood relatives have an increased risk of getting MS, they are still quite unlikely to develop the condition. More information about the role of genetics in MS is given in Chapter 2.

Reassuringly, the husbands, wives and adopted children of someone with MS are no more likely to get the condition than an unrelated person in the general population. It therefore appears that the increased risk of getting MS within family groups is not the result of a shared environment or similarities in lifestyles between family members.

Why is MS so common in some parts of the world compared to others?

A lot of scientific research has looked at the distribution of MS in different parts of the world. This is interesting both because it helps in the planning of services for people with MS, and also because it can give insights into the condition itself. Surveys that look at how common MS is in a particular area have to be interpreted cautiously, as many factors can affect the results.

Over much of the twentieth century, studies have shown increasing numbers of people with MS over time. A lot of the increases have been explained as being due to increased rates of diagnosis. For example, MS is more likely to be diagnosed when a new neurologist is appointed in an area where resources have previously been inadequate. MR scanning allows milder cases of MS to be diagnosed with more certainty and changes in the definition of MS can lead to more cases being identified. All of these factors mean that an *apparent* increase in the number of MS cases can be seen even when there has been no *real* change. The number of people with MS can also increase because of factors that have nothing to do with the number of new cases. For example, improvements in healthcare might lead to people with MS living longer, with the result that there will be more people with MS at any one time.

Having said all this, there do seem to be real differences in how common MS is in different parts of the world. One observation that has interested scientists is that MS seems to be more common the further you get from the equator. Even within the British Isles, MS is more common in the North and is especially common in the Shetland Islands and Orkney. In the USA, MS is more common in Northern and Western than in Central or Southern states. Why is this? Although at first sight, findings may appear to indicate there must be an environmental factor that depends on geographical latitude and longitude, a lot of the variation may be due to genetic differences in the people in these different regions. In the British Isles, for example, people of Celtic ancestry (who are found more frequently in the North) seem to be at greater risk of developing MS. In the USA, people of European – and especially Scandinavian – ancestry are more frequently seen to develop MS.

So do genetic factors, and ancestry, explain all of the differences in the rates of MS around the world? The answer is that they probably do not. A lot has been learnt from studies of people who migrate from areas where MS is common to areas where it is rare, or *vice versa*. Most of these studies suggest that if a person migrates after the age of about 15, their risk of developing MS stays the same as if they had not moved. People migrating at a younger age than 15 take on a risk that is between the rate in the country they have moved from and the one to which they have moved. This observation also seems to be true of the offspring of migrants. For example, MS is rare in Japan. The rates of MS seen in Japanese people living in Hawaii or California are significantly higher than for Japanese people who have stayed in

Japan, but nonetheless lower than in the rest of the Hawaiian and Californian populations. What does this mean? It seems that there must be environmental factors that modify the risk of MS, and that these factors are age-sensitive.

One frequently suggested theory is that there are infections – perhaps viruses – that are more common in places where MS is seen frequently. Exposure to such a viral infection before the age of 15 might prime the immune system in a way that causes the risk of developing MS later in life to be increased. Another suggestion is that higher rates of sunlight exposure help protect people from developing MS, possibly by increasing vitamin D levels in the body.

To summarise, MS is seen more commonly in some populations than others and the variability seen is likely to be due to an interaction between genetic and environmental factors.

Is MS becoming more common?

As we have discussed, MS may *appear* to be becoming more common for a number of reasons. In order to understand why this might be, it is important to know a little about how the number of people with MS is determined. Epidemiological surveys are used to find out how many people have MS in a certain geographical area at a particular time – this is known as the *prevalence* rate. When a survey is done for the first time not everyone with MS may be discovered and the survey may therefore underestimate the prevalence rate. If the survey is repeated a few years later, more people may be discovered because the investigators have become more experienced at finding people with MS. Indeed, they may discover people who actually had MS at the time of the first study but were not picked up at that time. Also, as the number of neurologists increases and access to MRI scanning improves, more people may be diagnosed with MS and at an earlier stage than in previous years. This is called *improved case ascertainment*.

These factors may explain how prevalence rates can increase over time, even though the actual number of people with MS may not have changed. Increased life expectancy of people with MS, due to specific treatments and interventions for MS and improved healthcare services in general, results in an increase in the number of people living with MS. This also contributes to an increase in prevalence rates over time, even though the number of people actually getting MS may not have changed. All these factors may explain, in part, why surveys done in countries with well-developed healthcare services tend to report higher prevalence rates for MS than those done in countries with poorer access to healthcare.

Are women at greater risk of developing MS than men?

Determining the risk of developing MS for any section of the population, or indeed for the population as a whole, depends upon on an accurate calculation of the numbers of people with MS within the population (*prevalence*) as well as the numbers of people diagnosed with MS during a given time period (*incidence*).

It has long been known that more women than men have MS. Studies of the *incidence* of MS in the UK over the last 10 years indicate that there is about twice as much chance of developing MS if you are female than if you are male. However, there is now some evidence emerging that the incidence in women is actually increasing; recent studies in both Canada and France show that the female to male ratio in MS has increased to 3:1. Although we don't know the reason for this increase, researchers think there must be an environmental factor influencing this change, and they are working hard to find out more about why this is happening.

Can children get MS?

They can, but it is very unusual. Only between 2 per cent and 5 per cent of people have their first attack of MS before the age of 16. It is important, therefore, that doctors test for a number of other conditions which are more in childhood and adolescence. These include inherited genetic, infective, inflammatory, blood vessel, nutritional, *metabolic* and cancerous causes – all of which will need to be ruled out before a diagnosis of MS can be made.

To help differentiate MS from these other conditions, the child's symptoms and signs will need to be considered, along with results of investigations such as blood tests, MRI and spinal fluid tests. A history of recent vaccination or infection, possibly associated with changes in behaviour, alteration in consciousness level or seizures (fits) might suggest disorders such as *ADEM* (acute disseminated encephalomyelitis).

2 | Types and course of MS

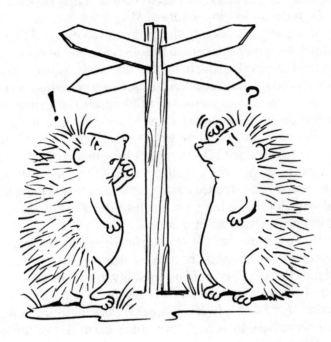

TYPES OF MS

This chapter explains the different ways in which MS can develop over time and to what extent we can currently predict a person's prognosis. It also explains some terms which may be confusing when you are reading about different types of MS.

How many different types of MS are there, and what distinguishes each of them?

MS can affect a person in a wide variety of ways and the features of the condition in one individual may be very different from those in another. Despite this, it is possible to identify different *types* of MS depending on the main characteristics of the condition and its change over time. In order to understand this, it helps to know a little more about the underlying nature of MS.

MS causes inflammation in the brain and spinal cord that comes and goes. Inflammation is caused by cells releasing substances which then attract more cells, which, in turn, themselves attract more in a cascade. Although similar processes are at work when you sprain your knee or a bee stings you on the arm causing the area to swell up, inflammation in MS does not cause the swelling to a significant degree, but nevertheless a number of cells which can cause damage to nerves are attracted into the brain or spinal cord. This inflammation causes symptoms if it affects a sensitive part of the central nervous system. This is called a *relapse* or an attack and the symptoms typically develop over a few days, stabilise over a few weeks and then slowly improve over weeks or months.

Whether a person partially or completely recovers from a relapse, depends upon the success of the body's natural repair mechanisms. A person may therefore accumulate disability in a step-wise fashion, as a result of relapses from which there has been incomplete recovery. The period of stability between relapses is called a *remission*. Relapses tend to occur less frequently over time because the underlying inflammation tends to diminish over the years.

MS also causes a slow process of nerve cell loss, called neurodegeneration. This may cause a slow deterioration in a person's condition that usually develops over many years and is called *progression*. Unfortunately, the exact nature of the link between inflammation and neurodegeneration is not fully understood.

The different types of MS are characterised by the patterns of *relapses* and *remissions* and/or *progression* over time – these depend on the extent of underlying inflammation, repair and neurodegeneration in the brain and spinal cord.

The term *relapsing-remitting MS* is used to describe the condition of a person who has relapses separated by periods of stability called remissions. The term *secondary progressive MS* is used when a person develops progression after a period of relapses and remissions. A person who develops this type of MS may also have relapses. The term *primary progressive MS* is used when a person starts with progression rather than relapses. If that person then has relapses, the term *progressive relapsing MS* is used.

These terms are generally accepted, understood and widely used. The new term *clinically isolated syndrome* (CIS) is not so well accepted but is often used to describe someone who has only had one attack or 'relapse'. If that person goes on to have another attack or relapse, or an MRI scan shows new inflammation, the term *relapsing-remitting MS* is then used. Another new term is *rapidly evolving MS*. This term is used by the National Institute for Health and Clinical Excellence (NICE) to identify a subgroup of people with relapsing-remitting MS who they

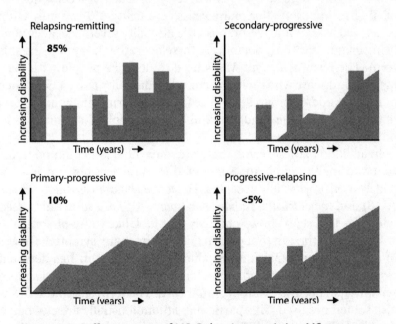

Figure 2.1 Different types of MS. Relapsing-remitting MS progresses to secondary progressive MS in around 50 per cent of patients after 10–15 years

have stated are eligible for treatment with *natalizumab* (Tysabri) on the NHS. The term is currently only used in this specific context.

There are some old terms that are now outmoded and no longer used. The term *chronic progressive MS* was previously used to describe a type of MS that is now known as either secondary progressive MS or primary progressive MS. The term *relapsing-progressive MS* has now been replaced by the term secondary progressive MS.

There are some other terms that are still used but are potentially misleading. The term *benign MS* is used to describe a person who has relapses and remissions with very good or complete recovery and no accumulation of disability over time as a result of relapses. However, so-called benign MS is probably best considered as a form of relapsing-remitting MS rather than as a separate disease type. This is because people with 'benign' MS may still develop disability as a consequence of progression even after many years of stability. MS can only truly be termed benign if a person has little disability several decades after being diagnosed. Many doctors are therefore rather wary of using this term. The term *malignant MS* is used to describe people with very aggressive disease who rapidly accumulate disability as a consequence of relapses and/or progression. The use of the term 'malignant' refers to the severity of the condition and does not imply it is cancerous in nature – it is not.

In addition to these terms, there are some other less common terms that you may read about. Some of these are very new, so not yet widely used or generally accepted. The terms *clinically absent syndrome (CAS)* and *radiologically isolated syndrome (RIS)* are sometimes used when an MRI scan shows changes that look like those of someone with MS even though that person does not have any symptoms of MS or signs of it on examination. That is, the MRI scan has detected evidence of underlying inflammation that has not yet affected a more sensitive part of the brain or spinal cord. The term *subclinical MS* is also sometimes used. This particular situation usually arises when a person has had an MRI scan for some unrelated reason (e.g. headaches) and the scan findings are entirely unexpected. If such a person then goes on to have a relapse or two, they may then be diagnosed with a clinically isolated syndrome (CIS) or relapsing-remitting MS.

Finally, it is important to appreciate that your doctor may be uncertain about the exact type of MS you have, or indeed whether you have MS at all. This is more likely to be an issue in the early stages of the condition: a more certain diagnosis may be established with further investigations or depending upon the change of your condition over time.

What will be the course of my MS?

The course of MS varies considerably from person to person and typically evolves over decades. Approximately 9 in 10 (90 per cent) people have relapses and remissions early in the course of their condition (relapsing-remitting MS) whereas the remainder experience progression from onset (primary progressive MS). Some people with relapsing-remitting MS may have very few relapses and complete recovery whereas others may have frequent relapses with incomplete recovery and accumulate disability as a consequence. Overall, recovery is complete or substantial in more than 4 out of 5 (80 per cent) relapses occurring early in the course of the condition. Also, the frequency of relapses tends to diminish over time. Nevertheless, 1 in 2 (50 per cent) people who start with relapsing-remitting MS go on to develop secondary progressive MS within 20 years from onset.

I am worried about what the future holds. Will I end up in a wheelchair?

Overall, 1 in 2 (50 per cent) people with relapsing-remitting MS need the use of a walking stick within 20 years from the start of their condition. This means 1 in 2 (50 per cent) people have *not* reached this particular milestone by that time. Indeed, some people may never develop significant walking difficulties. Unfortunately, it appears that those who start with primary progressive MS tend to reach this particular milestone a few years earlier than those who start with relapsing-remitting MS.

It is important to appreciate the figures quoted refer to what happens 'on average' to a *group* of people with MS and do not provide any useful insights into what may happen to an *individual* person at the time they are first diagnosed. Unfortunately, it is extremely difficult, if not impossible, to predict the future accurately for an individual person. The number of relapses someone has in the first few years is of quite limited predictive value and the extent to which a person recovers from early relapses is also not that helpful. In fact, it appears the most useful indicator of future disability is the onset of progression. Frustratingly, it is often quite difficult to identify the precise point at which a person enters the progressive stage of their condition. Once a person starts to progress, the rate of deterioration appears similar whether or not their condition started with relapses and remissions or progressed from onset.

Although MRI scanning is very useful in diagnosing MS it is not particularly helpful in predicting the onset of progression or future disability. Nevertheless, it is possible that novel forms of MRI scanning not currently in routine use may be shown to be helpful in this regard.

THE COURSE OF MS

Can you predict what the future holds for someone like me with MS?

The short answer is that, for an individual, we cannot predict the future with any accuracy. There are, however, some factors which are known to have an influence on prognosis.

The initial course of MS is the biggest factor that determines the outlook. If this is progressive, as in primary progressive MS, the prognosis is worse. Around 1 in 2 (50 per cent) people with an initially progressive course will need help walking within 10 years. Conversely, if the initial presentation is with relapsing-remitting MS, it will take around 20 years before 50 per cent of people will need help with walking.

Developing MS at a younger age is associated with slower accumulation of disability over time. This is largely or wholly explained by the observation that primary progressive MS tends to come on at an older age than relapsing-remitting MS. Once it has begun, the rate of progression in secondary progressive MS is similar to that of primary progressive MS. Some other factors can suggest a person may have a slightly better prognosis:

- Female sex – this may be because men are more likely than women to have primary progressive MS.

- Visual or sensory symptoms at onset – for example, optic neuritis, pins and needles or loss of feeling.

- Good recovery from early relapses.

- A long gap between first and second relapse.

On the other hand, weakness or poor coordination at onset suggest a worse prognosis.

Surprisingly, the number and size of abnormalities seen on early MRI scans, and lumbar puncture results, do not help a great deal in determining prognosis.

It appears that the *disease-modifying drugs* used in MS, including the beta-interferons (Avonex, Betaferon, Extavia, Rebif 22/44), glatiramer acetate (Copaxone) and natalizumab (Tysabri) may reduce the frequency, and possibly the severity, of relapses during the first few years of treatment. It is therefore possible these treatments may prevent some bad relapses that may otherwise have caused significant temporary disability. It is hoped these treatments, if started early in the relapsing-remitting phase of the condition, may delay progression or reduce the number of people developing secondary progressive MS and thereby reduce the number of people needing to use a wheelchair in later life. It is too early to tell at present whether or not this will be the case.

How often are people with MS given scans in order to keep track of the progress of MS?

In the UK, the majority of patients with MS are not routinely scanned once they have been diagnosed. There is no overall agreement between neurologists as to whether or not repeat scanning is appropriate or the specific circumstances in which this may be helpful. At present, most neurologists do not scan patients with MS after the diagnosis is confirmed unless the result of a further scan is likely to influence treatment decisions. For example, if your neurologist is thinking about whether to prescribe a disease-modifying drug or switch treatments (see Chapter 8), he or she may find it helpful to perform a further scan to see how active your MS is in order to support this decision. Occasionally, a repeat scan is required in order to determine whether or not you are eligible for a particular disease-modifying drug. This is currently the case in the UK for a new drug called natalizumab (Tysabri). If you develop an unusual neurological symptom which may or may not be related to your MS, or if the course of your condition departs from the expected pattern, your neurologist may choose to perform another scan in order to check if there is an alternative explanation for your problems.

I have relapsing-remitting MS. How likely am I to develop secondary progressive MS?

Studies have shown that when a group of people with relapsing-remitting MS are followed carefully over time, 50 per cent (1 in 2) of them will have entered the secondary progressive phase of the condition 20 years from the time of diagnosis. As the years go by, increasing numbers of people with relapsing-remitting MS will develop secondary progressive MS. However, up to 25 per cent (1 in 4) of people with relapsing-remitting MS may never go on to the secondary progressive stage of MS.

I have been told I have 'rapidly evolving MS' by my neurologist and that I may be suitable for treatment with natalizumab (Tysabri). What is 'rapidly evolving MS' and why am I 'suitable for treatment'?

The term rapidly evolving MS (REMS), was developed by the National Institute for Health and Clinical Excellence (NICE) to identify those people who they feel are most likely to benefit from, and therefore should be offered treatment with, natalizumab (Tysabri) on the NHS. It refers to patients with relapsing-remitting MS who have had 'two or more disabling relapses in one year' *and* 'one or more gadolinium-enhancing lesions on brain MRI or a significant increase in the number of T2 lesions compared with a previous scan'. The term REMS is currently used exclusively in this particular context and no other situation. Remember that people with REMS are usually also eligible for treatment on the NHS with the beta-interferons (Avonex, Betaferon, Extavia, Rebif 22/44) and glatiramer acetate (Copaxone) in accordance with Association of British Neurologists (ABN) guidelines (see Appendix 4).

Can you die from MS and, if so, how does it kill you and how soon?

Although MS can cause a wide variety of different symptoms and problems, it does not itself kill you. Most people with MS have a normal lifespan and die of non-MS related problems – dying *with* MS rather than *of* MS.

However, statistics do show that the average lifespan of someone with MS is a few years shorter than that of the general population. This doesn't mean that everyone with MS has a shorter lifespan, although it does mean that some people with more severe forms of MS are likely to experience a shorter lifespan than would otherwise be expected.

People who die with MS do so because of the complications of the disease rather than as a direct result of the condition itself. People with very advanced MS become particularly prone to infections – they may develop severe swallowing problems which can lead to food and saliva getting into the lungs resulting in repeated chest infections. Health professionals can do a great deal to manage problems such as these, but sometimes the MS gets so bad that, no matter what anyone does, the person seems to develop repeated infections. Eventually these just get too much and the individual dies as a direct result of this complication.

It is not possible to put a timescale on how quickly someone with advanced, severe MS may develop and succumb to infections in this way. Plenty of people in this position stay healthy for many years, although some can become very ill very quickly.

It is worth remembering that there is a lot more help and support available for people with severe MS today than there used to be. There is also greater understanding of the needs of people and their families who are in this situation. In addition to MS nurses, specialist neuro-rehabilitation teams and palliative care professionals are becoming increasingly involved in offering advice and support. There is also a range of other specialist individuals such as speech and language therapists, tissue viability nurses and community matrons.

3 | Genetic and environmental factors in MS

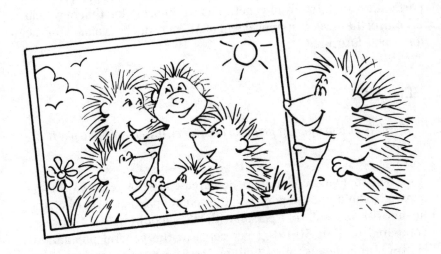

In this chapter we try to allay any concerns you may have about why you have developed MS and the risk of your children developing MS. We examine many environmental and lifestyle issues such as infections, vaccinations, diet, head injury and other trauma, and the relationship of MS to other illnesses.

The cause of MS is still unknown. Although there are significant variations in the distribution of people with MS throughout the world, research has failed to uncover any tangible evidence that there are any specific avoidable risks associated with the onset of the disease.

At present, it seems that the likelihood of developing MS is influenced by a combination of genetic and environmental factors. Studies of identical twins, where one or both has MS, offer what might be considered the most elegant way to investigate this theory. As a result of such investigations, it appears that genetic factors contribute 30–35 per cent and environmental factors 65–70 per cent to the risk of developing MS.

There does not seem to be one simple gene linked to MS and many different environmental factors may be involved. Despite the vast amount of research being carried out, and its rapid progress particularly in the study of genetic factors, information that may help to control the onset or management of MS may not be available for the forseeable future.

GENETICS

If MS is at least partly genetic, are my children going to get it too?

It is true that your children are at increased risk of getting MS compared to an unrelated person in the general population. In fact, the lifetime risk for a child of a person with MS is about 1 in 50 (2 per cent) compared to 1 in 500 (0.2 per cent) in the general population. However, this means that 49 out of 50 (98 per cent) children of an affected parent will *not* develop MS in their lifetime. Although there is some evidence that the son of an affected father is at even lower risk of getting MS when he grows up, this is uncertain. Unfortunately, if your spouse (husband or wife) also has MS, your children will have a relatively high chance of developing MS when they grow up (1 in 4 or 25 per cent). This is probably due to them getting a 'double dose' of the relevant genes from each parent. That said, it is important to appreciate this means 3 out of 4 of children (75 per cent) will *not* get MS.

If you have step-children or adopted children they are no more likely to get MS than someone in the general population (1 in 500 or 0.2 per cent). This is partly due to the fact that you are not related by blood, and therefore do not share any relevant genes. It also appears that any environmental factors (e.g. diet, viruses, lifestyle and climate) appear to act at a population level rather than within family groups.

Because MS tends to develop in young adulthood, you may have already decided whether or not to have children by the time you were diagnosed. That said, there is certainly no reason why you should not have children just because you have MS.

Have advances in genetics made it possible for people to have a test to see whether they are at risk of developing MS?

The short answer to this is 'no'. However, there are lots of interesting things that can be learnt about MS from the study of genetics.

The role of genes in MS has been studied extensively, and a great deal is now understood. We know that people of different ethnic origin have very different risks of developing MS, even when they live in the same region. This clearly points towards a role for genes in the development of MS. Similarly, descriptions of families where several people have MS also suggest that genes are likely to be important.

One of the most convincing demonstrations of the importance of genes comes from studying twins. The identical twin of a person with MS has a 1 in 4 (25 per cent) chance of having or developing MS themselves. The rate for non-identical twins is 1 in 50 (2 per cent). Identical and non-identical twins are likely to share the same upbringing, diet and other environmental factors. The fact that identical twins share exactly the same genes, whereas non-identical twins only have half (50 per cent) of their genes in common, is clearly very influential. Twin studies also show us that even when two people share exactly the same genes they will not necessarily both develop MS.

Five of my relatives, over three generations, have had MS. Are we a family with a special risk of MS, and should I ask for genetic counselling?

Close relatives of people with MS do have a higher risk themselves of having or developing MS. The risks are approximately 1 in 50 (2 per cent) for parents, 3 in 100 (3 per cent) for siblings, 1 in 50 (2 per cent) for children and 1 in 100 (1 per cent) for aunts, uncles, nephews and nieces of people with MS. When one particular family contains a number of people with MS, these risks are probably the explanation, although there may be some families that contain stronger genetic factors than those typically seen in people affected by MS.

Genetic counselling is not considered to be particularly useful for people with MS because blood tests are not accurate in predicting risk and the chances of having an affected child are relatively low.

CONNECTIONS WITH OTHER DISEASES

My MS flared up when I had an infection last year. The attack was particularly bad and I still haven't fully recovered. Could this have been the cause of the disease in the first place? If the attack was caused by an infection, should I avoid people or places where I might catch something?

It is not uncommon for someone who has had a relapse to be able to identify a recent infection and it is understandable why they may assume there is a link between the two events. However, it should be remembered that this apparent link could have been entirely coincidental. While it is true that studies show there may be a link between viral infections and relapses, the vast majority of people who have had infections do not go on to have relapses. Also, the design of many of these studies is flawed and a possible link has not been supported by MRI scan results. This apparent discrepancy is difficult to reconcile and reduces confidence in the studies' findings.

There have been many studies looking for evidence that particular infections may trigger the onset of MS but none have provided conclusive evidence of a causal link. Although there is some evidence implicating specific viruses, definite links have yet to be established. Indeed, the observation that people who are in close personal contact with someone with MS (e.g. spouses, adoptees and healthcare workers) are at no more risk of getting MS than the general population is very reassuring and provides no support for a possible contagious cause. It is important to appreciate that viruses are everywhere in the environment, and getting infections from time to time is unavoidable. Only a minority of such infections will actually produce recognisable symptoms and identifiable infections do not lead to relapses in the vast majority of cases. This means that, even though you have MS, it is not appropriate for you to avoid people or places, or to make any other specific lifestyle changes to avoid catching an infection.

I have read that some cases of MS are caused by infection. Is this true?

At the time of writing, a definite link between MS and a specific infectious agent has yet to be established. Indeed, it has not even been determined whether MS is related to an unusual response to a very common infectious agent or a number of different uncommon infections, or a common response to a rare infection. There has been a lot of research looking into the possibility that MS may be caused by a number of different viruses and bacteria. Studies have shown evidence of previous infections in a higher proportion of people with MS compared to those without MS. Other studies have found infectious agents, or antibodies to them, more frequently in the brains of people with MS compared to those without MS. Although these study findings may appear very convincing, there are a number of concerns, including the inability of a different group of scientists to reproduce the same result when an identical study is repeated. Some of the more convincing studies implicate infectious agents that are very common in the general population and this raises the interesting question as to why most people exposed to these infections do *not* develop MS.

A large body of work supports a link with the Epstein Barr virus (EBV) but, while this may turn out to be important, it is not proven and remains controversial. A number of viruses have been investigated over the years – from potential links with childhood illnesses (including measles, mumps and rubella), to a herpes virus HHV-6 and a retrovirus called 'multiple sclerosis associated retrovirus', but evidence has been inconclusive and, at times, contradictory. The bacterium *Chlamydia pneumoniae* has also been suggested as a possible candidate in the causation of MS.

Do infections cause relapses and if so, why?

Infections and other illnesses will naturally be expected to make people with MS feel more unwell than usual. As a result, symptoms that have been experienced before, or are present at the time, will often become more prominent. For example, a person with MS who is usually able to walk very slowly and unsteadily may find they cannot walk at all at the time of an infection and then improves once the infection has cleared. This sort of worsening of pre-existing symptoms is more likely to happen if the infection causes a rise in body temperature. If there are no new symptoms, then any deterioration at the time of an infection is unlikely to be a true relapse – it is sometimes known as a 'pseudo-relapse'. This is because a true relapse, which is caused by a new area of inflammation in the central nervous system, typically gives rise to new symptoms.

As well as the effects described above, it does seem to be the case (with the reservations mentioned earlier in this section) that true relapses are two or three times more likely to happen in the weeks just before and after viral infections. It is not clear why true relapses are more likely to happen around that time and there is no particular virus that has been shown to be implicated.

It is not clear whether viral infections make relapses happen by stimulating the immune system, or whether changes in the immune system that lead to a relapse also predispose people to getting viral infections.

Does MS weaken the immune system and make it more likely you may get colds and 'flu?

The common cold and influenza are both caused by viral infections. MS does not make the immune system weaker in the sense that it does not increase the risk of getting a virus.

However, treatment with immunosuppressive drugs including azathioprine, cyclophosphamide and mitoxantrone does weaken the immune system and increase the risk of infections. Furthermore, a new treatment called natalizumab (Tysabri) sometimes causes the reactivation of a latent virus causing a potentially very serious brain infection called *progressive multi-focal leukoencephalopathy* (PML). It is important to appreciate that these drugs are only offered to people if the benefits of treatment are considered to outweigh the side effects and risks. Needless to say, people receiving these drugs are carefully monitored and treatment is stopped if there is any cause for concern.

Conversely, it does appear that viral infections may trigger *some* true relapses in MS and that so-called 'pseudo-relapses' may occur at the time of viral infections.

Is MS linked in any way to other diseases?

The relatives of people with MS, and perhaps also affected people themselves, are more likely than the general population to get other conditions that are due to malfunctioning of the immune system. These so-called *autoimmune* diseases are thought to have features in common, so that the same environmental or genetic factors will increase the likelihood of a number of different conditions. Conditions that have reasonably convincingly been shown to be associated with MS include thyroid disease and psoriasis. There have also been links shown with Type 1 (early onset) diabetes, rheumatoid arthritis, ankylosing spondylitis, myasthenia gravis and inflammatory bowel disease, although the evidence that these autoimmune conditions are truly associated with MS is weaker.

One rare condition that is not autoimmune in mechanism, neurofibromatosis, has also been shown by some researchers to be associated with MS. It must be emphasised that most people with MS, and most of their close relatives, will not be affected by any of these conditions.

Is MS linked with cancer?

No. There is no direct link between MS and any form of cancer – a person with MS is no more or less likely to develop cancer than anyone else in the general population. However, it is not unusual for someone with MS to get cancer, particularly as they get older. This is because cancer is quite common and the risk of getting most forms of cancer increases with age.

However, some of the immunosuppressive drugs used in the treatment of MS, including azathioprine, cyclophosphamide and mitoxantrone, *are* associated with an increased risk of cancer. These drugs are not used routinely in MS and they are only offered when the benefits of treatment are considered to outweigh the side effects and risks.

The term *malignant MS* is used to describe a very aggressive form of the condition. The use of the term 'malignant' does not mean this form of MS is cancerous – it is not.

Is MS just a different and more severe form of another autoimmune disease, such as lupus?

MS is MS. It is not any other condition, and most people with MS will not have another major illness at the same time. Lupus, also known as *systemic lupus erythromatosis* or *SLE*, is an autoimmune condition that can affect the nervous system but it also causes skin, joint and kidney problems. Occasionally, people with lupus will have neurological problems that are similar to those seen in MS, but it is unusual for the two conditions to be confused.

ENVIRONMENTAL FACTORS

I have recently read that influenza injections can worsen MS. Should I avoid having a 'flu jab, or take my doctor's advice and have one?

It used to be recommended that people with MS should not have the 'flu jab because it was thought to increase the risk of a relapse. However, this is now known not to be the case.

Studies have shown that a vaccination does not increase the risk of a relapse or adversely affect the disease course. This evidence is so strong that it is included as a recommendation in the NICE (National Institute for Health and Clinical Excellence) guidelines about the management of MS and people with MS are now actively encouraged to have the 'flu jab each autumn.

It is now known that 'flu itself is far more likely to cause a relapse than receiving the vaccine, so the benefits of having the vaccine definitely outweigh any potential negatives.

I broke my arm a few weeks before the first symptoms of my MS developed. Do you think this could have caused my condition?

No. It is understandable that a person may link the onset of MS to a recent traumatic life event, such as an injury sustained in an accident, but this is purely coincidental. Studies have shown that accidental injury and the onset of MS occur together no more frequently than would be expected by chance. The overwhelming majority of medical opinion does not support any relationship between trauma and the onset of MS.

Doesn't it make sense that a head injury, or an injury near the brain or spinal cord, might have some adverse effect on MS?

It is entirely reasonable to think that a traumatic injury may cause a relapse or a progression of MS, particularly if it occurred to the brain or spinal cord. It is also tempting to think this may be due to disruption of the blood-brain barrier if the injury occurred at the same time as, and affected a part of the central nervous system that explained the symptoms of, the relapse. For example, a whiplash (neck) injury sustained in a road traffic accident shortly followed by an attack of partial myelitis (spinal cord relapse).

However, studies have shown that accidental injury and worsening of MS occur together no more frequently than would be expected by chance – that is, the two events are entirely coincidental. Indeed, the best available evidence does not provide any support for a causal link between recent trauma and relapses or progression in MS.

I have heard chronic mercury poisoning causes MS, so why aren't doctors doing more to warn people about the dangers of dental fillings?

It is true dental amalgam contains mercury and that it is currently used in the majority of fillings. It is also true that an excess of mercury in the body can result in damage to the central nervous system. It is therefore understandable why it has been claimed small amounts of mercury released from dental amalgam may cause MS, and why it has been suggested removal of dental amalgam may be therapeutic. However, there is no convincing scientific evidence that mercury causes MS, or that removal of dental amalgam is beneficial. Indeed, it is important to appreciate dental amalgam accounts for less than 10 per cent of all mercury ingested and that removal of fillings may actually result in a *greater* initial exposure to mercury than if they are left untouched. Furthermore, dental amalgam removal is expensive, time-consuming and may occasionally cause damage to teeth and nerves. Doctors do not recommend and usually discourage removal of dental amalgam for these reasons.

DIET

Is it possible that a bad diet causes MS?

A bad diet does not cause MS. That said, poor eating habits may contribute to some of the problems you may be experiencing as a result of having MS. For example, a bad diet resulting in weight gain may increase fatigue and exacerbate walking difficulties. A poor diet that causes weight loss and malnourishment due to lack of vitamins and minerals may contribute to fatigue and muscle weakness. Conversely, a healthy, well-balanced diet combined with exercise will help you to maintain your ideal weight, decrease fatigue and improve muscle strength. This will also be good for your general well-being.

I have heard food allergy may be to blame for MS. What are your thoughts on this?

There is currently no convincing scientific evidence that food allergy, or food intolerance, causes MS or makes it worse. Unfortunately, reliable testing for food allergy or intolerance is quite difficult because it requires a properly supervised exclusion diet. The whole process can be time-consuming and expensive. It is important to appreciate that even if it is shown you do have a food allergy or intolerance, it does not necessarily follow this is the cause of your condition.

If you are thinking about starting a special diet it is important to consider carefully how inconvenient or costly this will be and what you may gain from it. Some special diets (for example, gluten-free diets) exclude certain foodstuffs and may be rather unpalatable and difficult to stick to. You may find that following one of these diets turns out to be more troublesome than the symptoms it purports to alleviate.

WHY ME? IS IT MY FAULT?

I know that some people get MS, but why has it happened to me?

'Why me?' is often one of the first questions a person considers after they have been diagnosed with MS and it is one of the most difficult to answer. Unfortunately, the truth of the matter is that doctors do not really know why any particular person gets MS because the precise cause of the condition is unknown. Although it is true some people are more at risk of getting MS than others, it is still not possible to predict who will develop MS or explain adequately why some people with known risk factors get MS and others do not. It is very important to appreciate it is not your fault and that you are not to blame for developing MS. This is often difficult for some people to accept – these feelings are understandable and a normal part of the process of coming to terms with the diagnosis.

I know it sounds silly, but I often feel I've been punished for some bad things I did earlier in my life. I know it's not true, but why do I keep feeling like this?

It is normal to think of reasons why you may have developed MS. However, it is very important to understand that getting MS is not your fault – it is not the consequence of any wrongdoing or a judgement against you. It is certainly not a punishment. MS can affect 'good' and 'bad' people alike – it is not a moral arbiter.

It is entirely understandable that you may feel guilty or blame yourself, but any bad things you did in the past are completely unrelated to your MS. You should not keep these feelings to yourself. Just talking to a close friend, partner or relative about your concerns may be highly beneficial and help rid yourself of these feelings. If this doesn't help, it may be worth arranging to see a counsellor who will be able to spend time with you and help you talk through your concerns. Your GP or MS nurse may be able to refer you.

My first symptoms started when I was working hard for
promotion and exhausting myself. Could I have avoided MS by
slowing down a bit?

No. It is normal to link a life event with the onset of MS and conclude one may have caused the other when it did not. The fact you first developed MS when you were working hard is entirely coincidental. It is often not possible to avoid stress at work particularly if you are trying to demonstrate to your employers you are a suitable candidate for promotion. It is important to think positively about your own future and not disregard any of your life goals inappropriately just because you have MS. That said, if you have been overworking it may be worth thinking about your diagnosis as an opportunity to take stock of your current life situation and considering whether reorganising your work-life balance may be a good thing.

I am gay but my brother, who isn't gay, is completely healthy. Is
there a link between being gay and MS?

No. There is no link between your sexuality and your condition – it is simply a coincidence that you are gay and have MS. A gay person is neither more nor less likely to get MS than a heterosexual person.

I have always been teetotal, a non-smoker, eaten well and
exercised regularly. I know some people who have no respect for
their health but they seem perfectly OK. It just doesn't seem fair
– why did I get MS?

Unfortunately, keeping yourself fit and healthy is no guarantee against getting MS or any other condition for that matter. Although it is true some people who do not look after themselves may seem all right at present, they are actually putting their health at risk and storing up problems for themselves in the future. It is important to understand that your healthy lifestyle will help to reduce the risk of developing conditions such as diabetes, heart disease and cancer. It is therefore very important that you continue with your healthy lifestyle as it will help you to cope better with MS both now and in the years to come.

I have heard MS is a sexually transmitted disease – is this true?

No. It has been suggested that MS is a sexually transmitted disease and even that teenage-onset cases may be due to child abuse. Neither of these claims has any credibility and recognised authorities on the condition have vigorously refuted them. It is very regrettable that claims of this nature have been given a higher profile than they deserve and caused unnecessary distress and hurt to people with MS and their families.

4 | Diagnosis of MS

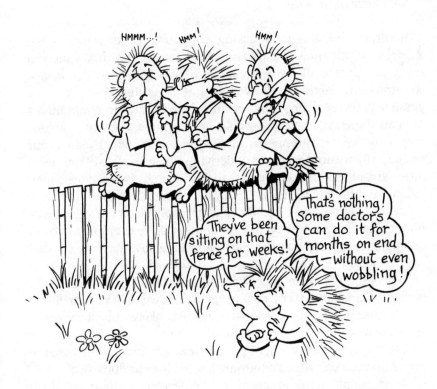

In this chapter, we consider when neurological symptoms might be a cause for concern and require further investigation, and what will happen when a neurologist assesses you. Some tips for getting the best from the consultation are included. We discuss some of the common tests involved in assisting with a diagnosis of MS, and what happens if you have had only one attack of symptoms suggestive of MS.

HOW WILL I KNOW?

I think I might have symptoms of MS. How do I know whether or not I have the disease?

Firstly, we should begin by asking why you think you have MS. Is it because you know or have read about someone with MS and you think you have similar symptoms? Perhaps it is because you have a well-meaning friend or relative who has suggested MS to you as a possible cause of your symptoms. It is true that some symptoms of MS can sometimes be non-specific. For example, they may include pins and needles, numbness or fatigue, all of which can occur temporarily without a serious underlying cause being to blame. Even other symptoms that can occur in MS – such as weakness, poor balance or blurring of vision – really need to persist to be of potential concern. Therefore any symptoms which only last a few minutes or hours or have gone the next day are not very likely to be due to MS. So an important secondary question is: how long do any symptoms that worry you last?

In general, the symptoms of a relapse or attack of MS tend to be persistent, and take several days to get to their worst before stabilising for another week or two. After this, there is likely to be a degree of spontaneous, sometimes incomplete, recovery. Compare this to any short-lived symptoms occurring over a few seconds, minutes or even hours and you can see that they are less likely to be due to MS.

Some people with progressive MS develop symptoms which gradually evolve over months to years, but again these are likely to be persistent, not temporary and short-lived.

How is MS usually diagnosed?

MS is mostly still diagnosed by an expert (for example a neurologist) based on your symptoms (what you tell them), and signs (what they find when they examine you) with support from other tests such as MRI scans and occasionally a spinal fluid test (lumbar puncture) and electrical tests, most commonly on the eyes (visual evoked response).

Even with advances in imaging the nervous system in detail such as MRI scans, the fundamental principle of diagnosing MS is for your neurologist to prove that there is spread (dissemination) of abnormalities of the central nervous system, for which there is no better explanation. This is because no test or group of tests is 100 per cent *specific* for MS (i.e. there is no test or group of tests that always gives a positive result in people with MS, and never does in anyone else). Sometimes, even after these assessments, it is still not possible for your neurologist to make a firm diagnosis of MS and he or she may need to keep you under review to see whether new symptoms develop, or may consider repeating your tests.

I am seeing a neurologist soon. What will he or she do?

Firstly, don't worry. Sometimes the symptoms can sound odd, for example, burning pain in an area that feels numb, electric shocks when you bend your neck forwards or problems with bowels, bladder or sexual function. Your neurologist will have seen lots of people with similar symptoms to yours and will be experienced in asking you about them.

Sometimes it is helpful to write down the dates of when your symptoms occurred, how long they lasted and whether they caused you any problems with work or home life.

It is always helpful to bring a relative or friend with you to your appointment. This is partly for moral support, partly to remind you of symptoms or attacks you may have forgotten to mention and also to help you remember what the neurologist says to you.

The neurologist will begin by asking you to describe the symptoms you have experienced. This will be to establish how many separate symptoms you have had, how quickly they came on and stayed and to what degree you recovered. He or she will then ask whether you have had specific symptoms, such as blurring of vision, double vision, slurring of speech, vertigo, bladder and bowel problems, stiffness or difficulty walking, and numbness or disturbed sensation such as tingling. You will then be asked about your general and previous health, medications taken, family history, alcohol intake, smoking history, occupation and social circumstances. This usually takes around 5–10 minutes.

Once the questions have been asked, the neurologist may watch you walk and check your balance before examining your vision. This will involve shining a light in your eyes, and checking your eye movements, facial strength and sensation. The neurologist may also examine your speech and tongue. He or she will then test your arms and legs for stiffness, strength, coordination, your reflexes (which involves tapping various tendons with a small instrument) and finally test your sensation to a sterile pin, vibration and joint position by moving the end of your finger and toe up or down with your eyes closed. Your neurologist will then decide whether further investigations are necessary.

At this point, the neurologist may express an opinion about the cause of your symptoms. This may take the form of reassurance that there is no evidence for concern, either on account of how you have described your symptoms or because of the examination findings. If you are concerned about the possibility of MS or other disorders you should feel free to raise these concerns, and your neurologist can address these directly. Your neurologist may feel unable to give a firm diagnosis at the time of the first consultation and wish to refer you for further tests such as an MRI scan, spinal fluid examination (*lumbar puncture*) and/or electrical tests such as *visual evoked responses*. Usually your neurologist will arrange an appointment a few weeks after the tests have been performed to discuss all of the results.

You can now request copies of all letters written about you and this can be helpful in ensuring that the information your neurologist has obtained from you is complete as well as for keeping up to date with the results of your tests. Some hospitals will ask you if you wish to have copies of correspondence copied to you: in other cases you may have to ask your neurologist.

TESTS

Can you tell me what tests I might have in order to be diagnosed with MS?

After your neurologist has spoken with you and examined you, there are a number of tests you might have to confirm or refute a diagnosis of MS.

You may be given some blood tests to rule out the possibility of other treatable conditions that can sometimes mimic MS. One of these is *systemic lupus erythematosis* (*SLE*) – a condition which can affect almost any part of the body and may include arthritis, rashes on sun-exposed areas, problems with eyes, nervous system and kidneys. Another is vasculitis – a series of disorders which cause swelling of the walls of blood vessels, narrowing the channel through which blood passes either slowing down or stopping its flow. As with SLE, many different parts of the body including the nervous system may be affected. Finally, vitamin B12 deficiency, which is more common in people with small bowel problems, can cause optic (eye) nerve problems, poor balance, changes in sensation in the feet and problems with memory and concentration.

Other tests that may be undertaken include an MRI scan, a lumbar puncture and a VER or visual evoked responses test. All of these are explained in more detail below.

What is an MRI scan?

An MRI (*Magnetic Resonance Imaging*) scan is a procedure that uses magnetic fields to take detailed pictures of internal organs. Many people with suspected MS will have an MRI scan of their brain and sometimes the spinal cord. Sometimes, an injection of dye (*gadolinium* – see answer to the following question) is given to gain additional information from the scan, but this is usually not needed. Your doctor will be able to tell you whether an injection may be needed before you go for your scan. It is possible that your neurologist may wish to repeat the scan or arrange other tests if the results are inconclusive.

Because MRI scans involve magnetic fields, the radiographer will run through a list of questions before you have the scan to check that it is safe for you to enter a magnetic field. They will ask you to remove any metal objects including jewellery and piercings, watches and credit cards.

If there is any chance you may be pregnant, you should tell your doctor in advance or the radiographer before the scan. Although there is no conclusive evidence that having an MRI is harmful to a baby, the technique has not been available long enough for us to be sure. So, unless your doctor still feels the benefit to you of having a scan at that point outweighs the potential risks, the scan should be postponed until after you have given birth.

Usually you cannot have an MRI scan if you have a pacemaker or cochlear (ear) implant as the magnetic field may interfere with their function. Longstanding replacement joints are usually OK. If you have any concerns, speak to the radiographer *before* the scan.

The scanners are very noisy (they make a banging sound) and can be claustrophobic. You can't take anyone in with you and you will need to keep still for 10–15 minutes. It is important to follow the radiographer's instructions and keep as still as possible. You can ask the radiographer to talk to you via headphones and ask for music to help you relax. If you are very nervous, a sedative may be given. This may need to be arranged beforehand with your doctor and you will not be allowed to drive home afterwards.

What do MR scans tell you?

Magnetic resonance imaging (MRI) scans of the brain and/or the spinal cord can be used for a number of aspects of management in MS, including supporting a clinical diagnosis, and assessing people for, and monitoring their response to, disease-modifying treatment. It can also be used to identify other illnesses that may mimic MS.

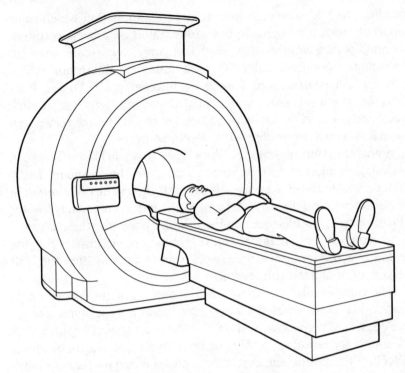

Figure 4.1 Having an MRI scan

MRI scan findings can be used to support a diagnosis of MS in people who have had appropriate clinical symptoms and in whom the neurologist has found suggestive clinical signs. MRI scans are now routinely used in the investigation of MS. However, it is important to understand MRI scanning is not a substitute for, but is complementary to, the clinical assessment by a doctor. That said, if the MRI scan of brain and spinal cord is entirely normal, the clinical diagnosis should be questioned and repeat scanning after an interval or other tests may be needed

The brain is divided into *grey matter* which contains the origin of nerve cells, the cell bodies, and *white matter* which contains the tendrils (processes) of nerve which are normally surrounded by myelin. The MRI scan can show areas of inflammation which show up as white dots (lesions) in the white matter on a background of normal-looking white matter, which looks grey on the scan. New MRI techniques are demonstrating that areas of the brain which previously appeared normal are in fact affected by MS. This explains why the appearances on your recent MRI scan may not closely match your current level of disability and also may not change very much even if you improve or deteriorate significantly.

Sometimes your neurologist may suggest that you have a dye called gadolinium injected into the vein in your arm. This would normally remain within the bloodstream; however if there is any disruption in the *blood-brain barrier* (BBB) which, as the name suggests, separates the brain from the bloodstream then the dye flows into these areas of inflammation, 'enhancing' them. This enhancement implies that the lesion is acute and only a few weeks old. After this time the BBB repairs itself and the enhancement fades.

The number, size, location and orientation of these white dots (lesions) can then be used to imply whether or not the abnormalities are consistent with a diagnosis of MS. The main reason for this is that although appearances on MRI can be suggestive of MS, for example, affecting the brainstem, cerebellum and the corpus callosum (see Figure 1.1 at the beginning of this book), they are not usually totally conclusive, especially in people over 50. This is why the result of an MRI must be considered in context with the symptoms you have experienced and the clinical signs found by the neurologist who examined you. For example, white dots can also occur as part of the normal ageing process as well as in people with high blood pressure and other risk factors for stroke. An MRI of the spinal cord can be helpful in this case as it is much less likely that white dots will occur in the spinal cord due to stroke disease.

People with primary progressive MS have fewer white dots, on average, on their scans than those with relapsing-remitting MS and a combined scan of the brain and spinal cord can again be helpful. It is more likely that other tests (such as VER and lumbar puncture) may be needed to confirm diagnosis in this situation.

An Expert Panel of Neurologists has revised the diagnostic criteria for MS. These are known as the McDonald Criteria, and more detail about them is given in Appendix 3.

My doctor says I need a lumbar puncture. What exactly is going to happen?

A *lumbar puncture*, also known as a *cerebrospinal fluid* (CSF) examination, is one of the tests often used in the diagnosis of MS.

Lumbar puncture is usually performed as a day case. It is sensible to arrange for someone to drop you off and pick you up so that you do not have to drive and can take it easy for the rest of the day. Your hospital may have a specific lumbar puncture information sheet which will explain the procedure in more detail. A lumbar puncture involves you either lying down on your left side and curling up or sitting upright and forward, as shown in Figure 4.2. Follow the instructions the doctor gives you to bend your spine as best as you can as this will help to make the lumbar puncture easier to perform. Remember, if at any stage you wish the doctor to stop temporarily, you should ask him or her to do so, and if you want to move for any reason (for example, if you have cramp) ask the doctor first if it is safe to do so.

Initially, your skin is cleaned with a sterilising solution which may feel cold. Then a local anaesthetic is given to numb your lower back and the doctor will wait a few minutes for this to work. As a result, the thin hollow spinal needle should not feel sharp when it is carefully inserted, although you may still feel a pressure or pushing sensation. Occasionally, you may get a shooting pain, either in your back or down one leg, which is due to irritation of a nerve – let the doctor know and he or she will stop and re-position the needle.

A small quantity of spinal fluid is collected from the needle. This is tested for any presence of infection, protein content, sugar levels and the presence of *oligoclonal bands* (OCBs – see Figure 4.3) A count of the numbers of white and red blood cells in the spinal fluid is also made.

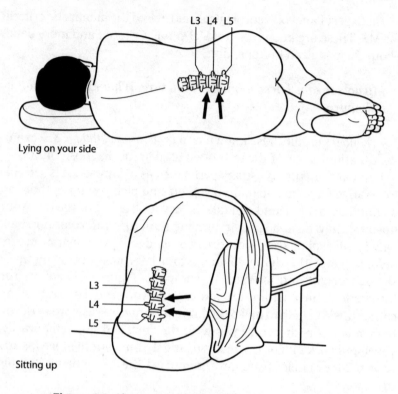

Lying on your side

Sitting up

Figure 4.2 Alternative positions for a lumbar puncture

OCBs are types of proteins that are made by the immune system in response to a trigger. By comparing your spinal fluid and blood, it is possible to see whether the oligoclonal bands are present in the spinal fluid alone (and not the blood). If so, this suggests the immune system has been activated in the brain and/or the spinal cord. Although oligoclonal bands provide support strong for the diagnosis, being present in over 90 per cent of people with MS, they may also be found in a variety of other conditions, some of which can mimic MS. Once again, therefore, their presence or absence is but one aspect of the overall picture that your neurologist considers when making a diagnosis of MS.

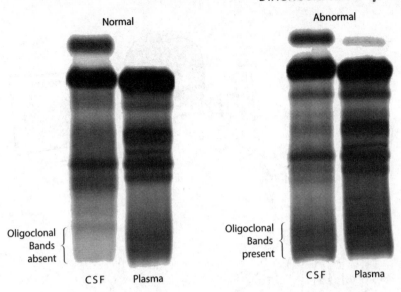

Figure 4.3 Oligoclonal bands (OCBs)

Following a lumbar puncture, you may sometimes have a little backache or headache. This will usually subside. We recommend that you lie flat for a period of time following a lumbar puncture and make sure that you are not dehydrated by drinking plenty of fluids, although the evidence behind these recommendations is sparse. It is sensible to have plans in place so that you can rest for the remainder of the day after a lumbar puncture should you find the need to do so. Very occasionally, people do have prolonged symptoms after a lumbar puncture. If you have the opportunity to reschedule your work and home commitments just in case you do have a prolonged headache or vomiting, for example, this can be helpful. You should contact your doctor for advice in these circumstances.

What is a VER?

Visual evoked response (VER) is a test that measures the speed of electrical conduction. This usually involves an eye test, where you

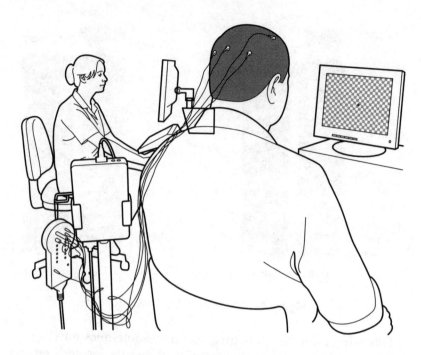

Figure 4.4 Procedure for recording the visual evoked response (VER). The patient looks at the television screen.

sit in front of a chequerboard on a television screen (see Figure 4.4). It is not a painful procedure. In MS, because the lagging around the nerves (myelin) has been damaged, the electrical nerve impulses travel more slowly along the nerves and the tests can demonstrate this. Once again these abnormalities are not specific to MS.

Very rarely, your neurologist may consider performing other electrical tests on your ears, or possibly a test on your spinal cord involving the placing of electrodes on your big toe, lower back and head. But these have largely been replaced by the widespread use of MRI scans and are only used in exceptional circumstances, for example, if you couldn't have an MRI scan because of a pacemaker or other reason.

Why do I need so many different tests?

As we mentioned earlier, there is no test or group of tests that can demonstrate a positive result for MS and is negative in all other situations. Blood tests, MRI scans, lumbar punctures and VERs all provide different sorts of information about underlying pathology (for example, VER is the only way to show demyelination). An MRI is sometimes sufficient, but other tests may be necessary, and all tests may need to be repeated if, for example, clinical presentation is not typical.

When diagnosing MS, why do neurologists scan only the head? Why not the spine as well?

You are right in implying that MS is a disorder of the central nervous system, which includes the brain and spinal cord. So it is entirely logical to ask why neurologists sometimes only scan your brain. The simple reason is this: when an MRI scan of the brain is clearly abnormal with sufficient numbers of white dots or plaques in regions typically affected by MS, then there is little additional information to be gained from an additional MRI scan of the spine.

So, if your symptoms and signs are attributable to a disorder affecting the brain, and your brain scan demonstrates clear-cut changes consistent with MS (perhaps with supportive evidence from spinal fluid and/or VER tests) then scanning your spine, whether or not it shows the white dots or plaques of MS, is not going to change the way your neurologist manages your condition.

If your symptoms and signs point towards the spinal cord as being affected and your neurologist considers MS a possible diagnosis, you are likely *also* to have a brain scan as this can provide important diagnostic and prognostic information about whether it is normal or abnormal. This can be important, for example, when you have a first attack suggestive of MS (called a *clinically isolated syndrome*), or in people with primary progressive MS where the symptoms can get gradually worse over a long period of time.

Where an MRI scan of your spine is useful is if your brain scan shows abnormalities but these (and perhaps your symptom or signs) are not typical of MS, or if you are over 50 and in particular if you are at higher risk for problems with arteriosclerosis or stroke (for example, because of heavy smoking, high cholesterol, diabetes mellitus or previous angina or heart attack). In these cases the spinal cord is less commonly affected by poor blood flow than the brain, so a normal spinal MRI would point away from an inflammatory cause for your symptoms such as MS and more towards a problem with blood flow. On the other hand, an abnormal spinal MRI with white dots or plaques would suggest MS despite these other confounding factors. Your neurologist may also wish to use the other supporting tests such as lumbar puncture and visual evoked responses (VER).

I have looked up the diagnosis of MS on the Internet and found a reference for the McDonald Criteria. What are these?

The McDonald Criteria are named after Professor Ian McDonald, the Chairman of the original group of MS experts who published their guidelines for the diagnosis of MS in 2001. These were revised in 2005 (see Appendix 3), and are the latest attempt to distil the essential requirements for a diagnosis of MS. It is important to be aware that these are consensus guidelines for the diagnosis of MS in adult, western people. They may not apply to children or to non-caucasian people.

Although the McDonald Criteria are helpful in providing a framework for diagnosis, consultant neurologists use their experience to weigh up all of the information they have about an individual patient's symptoms, clinical signs and test results and any unusual features which might suggest an alternative diagnosis. Therefore, they may conclude that the most likely cause for a person's symptoms is still MS, even though the McDonald Criteria may not be met in full. Given that no combination of symptoms, signs and test results occurs only in MS, there may be occasions when a person with an alternative diagnosis (such as *sarcoidosis* or *systemic lupus erythematosus*) may fulfil the McDonald Criteria. This emphasises the importance of the neurologists' experience in weighing up all of the information they have about an individual case before reaching a diagnosis.

Appendix 3 shows various scenarios in table form, indicating how MRI scans and other tests can be used to help in reaching a diagnosis of relapsing-remitting MS.

I have had a single attack of optic neuritis and I have been told that my brain scan has shown three 'lesions'. My neurologist says that I have had a 'clinically isolated syndrome'. What is a clinically isolated syndrome and what is my risk of developing MS?

A clinically isolated syndrome (CIS) is a single attack of inflammation affecting the brain or spinal cord but without a history, or evidence on examination of any previous episodes.

The three commonest clinically isolated syndromes are optic neuritis, disorders of the brainstem or cerebellum, and inflammation in the spinal cord (partial myelitis).

Optic neuritis is inflammation of the optic (eye) nerve which arises as a stalk on each side of the front of the brain. Some people wake up with blurred vision which typically gets worse over a few days. You may notice that colours, especially reds and blues, become less intense when you compare looking at an object with your normal eye. You can feel an aching or stabbing pain on eye movement. Sometimes you may notice the centre of your vision is reduced and that you have to move your head 'to look around' this gap in vision to see things properly. Typically, people regain enough vision in the affected eye to be able to read a number plate from a distance as necessary for passing a Driving Test.

The brainstem connects the brain to the spinal cord. The cerebellum lies behind it at the base of the skull and there are many connections between the brainstem and cerebellum. Therefore, any disease which affects one can disturb the function of the other. MS can affect both. Typical symptoms include double vision, slurring of speech, lack of co-ordination and imbalance.

Spinal cord disease typically causes a combination of weakness and disturbed sensation of the legs and sometimes the arms, disturbance of bladder, bowel and sexual function and sometimes either a tight band or hypersensitive patch around the midriff.

Long-term follow-up studies of 15 to 20 years after the onset of a clinically isolated syndrome (CIS) have shown that if a baseline brain MRI scan is *normal* except for the lesion that caused the CIS, then around 1 in 5 people will have a second clinical attack in 20 years, that is develop MS. If the baseline MRI scan is abnormal and shows additional lesions, then 4 in 5 of these people will have a second attack within 20 years. Therefore, although MRI scans are helpful for prognosis, again they do not accurately predict in everyone whether their CIS will progress or not.

I had an MRI scan for investigation of bad migraine. My GP said that the report says it shows changes 'typical of MS'. He referred me to a neurologist who said that I have a 'radiologically isolated syndrome'. I didn't understand this. What does he mean?

MRI scans are much more widely available than they used to be. Indeed, GPs can now organise them, so you can have a scan without necessarily seeing a hospital specialist. One consequence of this is that it is now more likely that a number of unexpected and sometimes incidental findings will be demonstrated that would otherwise have not come to light before you were referred to a specialist.

There is now a considerable number of people, like yourself, who have had an MRI scan for other reasons, which seems to show changes typical of those we see in MS, but without any previous history of consistent clinical symptoms, or any clinical signs when you are examined by a neurologist. This is a radiologically isolated syndrome, clinically absent syndrome or subclinical MS.

In one study of such people over five years of follow-up, MRI scans demonstrated new changes in three quarters and clinical attacks in about one third. At present, doctors do not prescribe disease-modifying drugs routinely to patients in this situation. However, you can expect to be kept under review and if you have neurological symptoms affecting your brain and/or spinal cord then you may have developed a clinically isolated syndrome (see the previous answer). A further attack would suggest the development of relapsing-remitting MS.

RECEIVING THE NEWS

Communicating any diagnosis that might affect a person's life is never easy. More information about the relationships between you and your healthcare team can be found in Chapter 7.

My doctor says that I 'probably' have MS. What does that mean and why the lack of certainty?

As explained above, there is no test or group of test results occurring only in MS, so therefore the diagnosis is based upon a combination of your symptoms, clinical signs found by your doctor and test results. A diagnosis of MS depends upon proving that there is spread or dissemination, with at least two lesions (damage to a specific area of the brain or spinal cord) which have occurred at different times, with no better explanation. There have been several attempts to produce generally accepted diagnostic criteria that grade the certainty of a diagnosis of MS, particularly when your neurologist cannot demonstrate two different lesions separated in time. In 1983, Dr Poser published criteria to help define the certainty of the diagnosis of MS, mainly for research purposes. Poser used the terms 'definite' and 'probable MS' in these situations. The most recent criteria (the Revised McDonald Criteria 2005 – see Appendix 3) do not use the terms: patients either have MS or they do not. Again, they are helpful for people conducting research in MS. In real life situations, however, although you may not fulfil all of the criteria strictly to the letter, based upon all of the assessments listed above the most likely explanation for your symptoms, signs and test results is MS. Your neurologist will use his or her experience to reach a pragmatic judgement as to whether or not a diagnosis of MS can be made.

> *I believe that my neurologist knew that I had MS several months before she actually told me. Why did she not tell me when she knew?*

It is possible that your neurologist felt that the diagnosis of MS was likely but she did not have enough evidence from your symptoms, examination findings or tests such as MRI scanning to be certain. A misdiagnosis of MS can be very damaging. Your neurologist may have been waiting for further evidence of MS to declare itself; such as you experiencing further symptoms, or new signs when she examined you, or new abnormalities on repeat tests before giving you the diagnosis.

> *My neurologist told me bluntly and clearly that I had MS, but he didn't offer any hope for the future at all. I had to find out what I could do for myself. Is this usually the case?*

No, this isn't how people are usually told they have MS, and nor should it be. We are sorry to hear you have had such a negative experience.

There is a wide range of reaction to a diagnosis of MS. For some people it can bring tears of relief after having been either told or made to feel that they were imagining their symptoms. For others, it can seem like a death sentence, something that takes a long time to come to terms with. Most people have a reaction that is somewhere in between.

There are a number of sources of information and support for people newly diagnosed with MS. Your neurologist and/or MS nurse will be able to answer your questions. You may be invited to a course for people with a new diagnosis of MS so that you can share your experiences with others who are in the same situation and know that you are not alone.

There are also two excellent patient groups: the MS Society and the MS Trust, both of which provide a wealth of information, help and practical support to people with MS, their carers and families. There are a number of other resources listed in the Appendices at the back of this book. In this day and age, no one should have to face the challenges of MS on their own.

To my surprise, when my neurologist gave me my diagnosis at the hospital several people 'sat in' on it. I thought it should have been just my husband and myself and the neurologist. Why was that?

If people do not introduce themselves, you should always ask who they are and, if you prefer, request they do not sit in on your consultation. However, a diagnosis of MS can lead to a number of emotions as we have discussed. It can be viewed as breaking bad news. It is likely that an MS Specialist Nurse or other members of the MS multidisciplinary team were sitting in on your consultation because it was helpful to know exactly what was said to you and what your reaction and that of your husband was to the news of the diagnosis. People often do not take in much information after a diagnosis is given and therefore we expect that the other people sitting in will need to contact you after the dust has settled a little, and be prepared to answer your questions and repeat some of the information that you may have forgotten in the heat of the moment.

CONDITIONS SOMETIMES CONFUSED WITH MS

I have read on the internet that Hughes' syndrome can sometimes be confused with MS. What is this?

Hughes' syndrome or antiphospholipid (AL) syndrome is a disorder which can lead to blood clots in both arteries and veins. Although it can sometimes be considered as a potential mimic of MS, usually the different clinical features are characteristic and blood tests can be helpful in distinguishing the conditions. In antiphospholipid syndrome, antibodies are made against phospholipid which is part of the surface of cell membranes. Possible consequences may be recurrent miscarriages or premature birth due to eclampsia (fits), stroke or deep vein thrombosis in the legs or elsewhere and *pulmonary embolism*. Some people may also have a low platelet count and a mesh-like rash called livedo reticularis. Antiphospholipid syndrome can occur on its own, or in conjunction with other disorders such as systemic lupus erythematosus. It is important to note that a diagnosis of antiphospholipid syndrome requires the occurrence of a blood clot or miscarriage or premature birth due to eclampsia (fits) and two positive blood tests at least three months apart. Therefore, if you have not had one of these clinical events, but have a single positive blood test, that in itself does not confirm a diagnosis of antiphospholipid syndrome. In the vast majority of cases there should be no confusion between antiphospholipid syndrome and MS if a detailed assessment is undertaken.

I've heard that a condition called Devic's disease can be mistaken for MS. How do I know whether I've got it?

Devic's disease (also known as neuromyelitis optica or NMO) is another potential 'MS mimic'. It is a condition that causes repeated relapses affecting either the optic nerves (optic neuritis) or spinal cord (transverse myelitis) and is therefore easily confused with

MS. However, it does not cause any of the other sorts of relapses encountered in MS. Also, the relapses in Devic's disease are typically much more severe than those in MS, and recovery is usually incomplete or negligible. As a consequence, people with Devic's disease tend to accumulate disability as a consequence of bad relapses rather than because of progression of their condition.

It is very important to distinguish Devic's disease from MS because it is treated differently. The disease-modifying drugs most often used in MS (the beta-interferons and glatiramer acetate) are at best ineffective in Devic's disease, and in the case of beta-interferon potentially harmful. Fortunately, tests can help separate these two conditions – a blood test for an antibody called NMO-IgG may confirm Devic's disease, MRI scanning may reveal abnormalities not usually encountered in MS and a lumbar puncture may also be helpful.

5 | Symptoms of MS

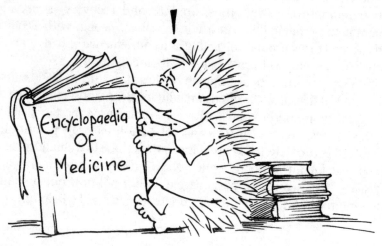

There are many symptoms encountered in MS. They may be temporary and mild, or more persistent and troublesome. This chapter talks about MS symptoms in general. More detailed information on specific problems encountered in MS are given in later chapters. Symptoms of MS can, for example, include problems with:

- Bladder and bowels (Chapter 12)
- Pain and sensations (Chapter 13)
- Cramps and spasticity (Chapter 13)
- Fatigue, cognition and mood (Chapter 14)
- Mobility, balance and tremor (Chapter 15)
- Speech and swallowing (Chapter 16)
- Eyesight and hearing (Chapter 17)
- Sexual function (Chapter 18).

Symptom management in MS is often challenging. Symptoms may be wide-ranging and variable to the extent that a variety of strategies is often required. These may include lifestyle changes, drug therapies, psychological or counselling support, physiotherapy, speech and occupational therapies, use of equipment, environmental modifications and, in some cases, surgery. Many symptoms may involve more than one of these interventions and different health care professionals. The main concern for all those involved in managing your symptoms, including you and your family, is to find an appropriate balance between all the therapies, especially when several symptoms occur at the same time.

I know that many symptoms are linked to MS. Are there any particular ones that may catch me by surprise?

MS is a condition that, by its nature, causes symptoms that may catch you by surprise. You may have relapses and these tend to occur on an unpredictable basis, often without warning. These relapses can cause a variety of symptoms, the nature of which depends upon the part of the central nervous system affected (see Chapter 5). You may also find some of the symptoms you experience surprising because they are wrongly considered not to be a feature of the condition or are embarrassing and therefore under-reported. These sorts of 'hidden' symptoms include fatigue, pain, bladder and bowel problems, and sexual difficulties (see Chapters 14, 13, 12 and 18).

What are the usual symptoms of MS and how would I recognise them?

MS may cause a variety of different symptoms. Although many are easily recognisable by their nature, others are much less characteristic and may have other causes. It is very important for you to be familiar with the sorts of symptoms that are typical of MS and the others that are more non-specific in nature. This knowledge will enable you to develop some expertise in the management of your own condition and as a result you will have a much clearer idea of where to seek further advice and help. It is fair to say that a fully informed, so-called 'expert patient' is in a much better position to make appropriate use of available services than those who do not fully understand their own condition.

An MS relapse (or attack) causes symptoms, the nature of which depends upon the part of the brain or spinal cord (central nervous system) affected by inflammation. For example, a relapse involving the eye (optic) nerve may cause blurred vision and pain in one eye (optic neuritis), one affecting the brainstem may cause double vision, slurred speech, clumsiness and/or unsteadiness (brainstem relapse), and one in the spinal cord may cause leg weakness and/or bladder problems (partial or transverse myelitis). Typically, the symptoms a person may experience in a relapse increase over a few days, stabilise for a few weeks and then improve over a period of weeks to months.

Other typical symptoms encountered in MS may last only a brief period of time but recur repeatedly. For example, *Uhthoff's phenomenon* refers to temporary symptoms that usually occur during exercise or in hot conditions. A typical example would be a temporary blurring of vision in one eye – often in an eye previously recovered from optic neuritis. *Lhermitte's phenomenon* refers to a brief wave of tingling or numbness affecting the arms or legs that may occur on bending your neck forward – this typically occurs during or following a relapse affecting the spinal cord in the neck (partial or transverse myelitis). *Trigeminal neuralgia* causes severe electric shock or sharp, shooting facial pains that typically last for seconds only, but may recur very frequently. It may be triggered by the slightest touch, eating or facial movement. So-called 'tonic spasms' may cause brief spasms or tingling pains in the arms or legs.

Some other symptoms that occur in MS are more persistent or can 'wax and wane' on a day-to-day basis. For example, fatigue is very common in MS and sometimes very troublesome. Pain is also common and bladder, bowel and sexual problems are probably under-reported in MS. No symptoms are specific to MS, and may have other causes.

What sort of symptoms will I start to experience now that I have been diagnosed with MS?

The period around diagnosis is always difficult, not least because it marks the beginning of a steep learning curve. Suddenly tiny things which you may have hardly noticed before gain new significance, and it can feel as though you are being bombarded with lots of different symptoms and also lots of new information. This is a very normal and common way to feel. You will soon learn which symptoms are important and which are not of great significance. Your MS nurse, if you have one, can be a big help in this process.

Always remember that receiving a diagnosis of MS does not change the symptoms you have been experiencing. It does mean, however, that will you know what you are dealing with and this knowledge will put you in a much better position to access the appropriate help, support and treatment you need to help manage these symptoms.

Everyone with MS is different and it is not sensible to give an exhaustive list of possible symptoms you may experience in the first year or so after diagnosis. Individuals vary so much that it is impossible to generalise. What we can say, however, is that most people will continue to experience the same sort of problems they were coping with before being diagnosed. If you can arrange to speak with your MS nurse or neurologist you may find that they are able to give you a better idea of what to expect.

Something important to be aware of in the period following diagnosis is that some people do become anxious and depressed. Again, this is a fairly common reaction to receiving a diagnosis of MS. If you, or people close to you, are worried that you may be getting very low in mood, make an appointment to talk to your MS nurse or GP. They can help you deal with symptoms like these and you may be surprised to find how much better you feel once anxiety and/or depression are being effectively treated.

Is it true that no two people with MS have exactly the same symptoms?

Yes and no! Although it is true that no two people share the exact same combination of symptoms it is not unusual for two people to have some symptoms in common. For example, a person may have blurred vision in one eye, leg weakness and some difficulties with bladder control due to previous attacks of optic neuritis and partial myelitis (see Chapter 6). Another person may have blurred vision in one eye, slurred speech and clumsiness due to a previous attack of optic neuritis and a brainstem relapse (see Chapter 6). These two people have one symptom in common – blurred vision in one eye – and others they do not share. By the same token, two patients may have the same sorts of symptoms but to different degrees. For example, one person may have very troublesome fatigue that affects their day-to-day life and some mild unsteadiness that is not too much of a problem, whereas another person may have mild fatigue together with considerable walking difficulties.

6 | Relapses

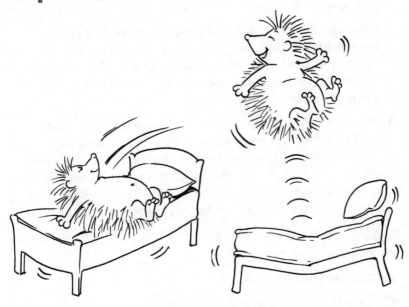

In this chapter we consider the difference between symptoms of MS and the characteristics of a 'relapse'.

I have heard people talk about relapses of MS. What does that mean?

In order to explain what a relapse (also known as an attack, exacerbation, bout, or episode) of MS, is it is important to understand a little about the underlying nature of the condition. MS causes inflammation in the brain and spinal cord (central nervous system) that comes and goes. This inflammation only causes immediate symptoms if it affects a sensitive part of the central nervous system. The nature of these symptoms depends on the area of the central nervous system that is affected. For example:

- Inflammation of the optic nerve typically causes reduced vision in one eye and pain made worse by eye movement. This is called *optic neuritis.*

- Inflammation in the part of the brain that controls eye movements, balance and coordination (brainstem and cerebellum) may cause double vision, 'jumping' vision, vertigo (spinning sensation), clumsiness or unsteadiness. This is called a *brainstem relapse.*

- Inflammation in the spinal cord may cause weak legs and walking difficulties, numbness, tingling or problems with bladder and bowel control. This is called partial or transverse *myelitis.* Occasionally, a person with this sort of attack may also develop an odd feeling down their back when they bend their neck forwards known as Lhermitte's phenomenon.

The symptoms of a relapse tend to:

1. Develop over a few days;
2. Stabilise for a few weeks;
3. Then improve over weeks or months;
4. Be followed by a period of stability (a remission).

The severity of relapses may vary considerably: some may be mild with complete recovery whereas others may be severe with only partial recovery. The frequency of relapses may also vary – one person may have an attack and then no further relapses for many years whereas another person may have relapses every few months. Overall, people tend to have fewer relapses as time goes by. This is because there is usually less inflammatory activity in people with longer-standing MS than in the earlier stages of the condition.

It is important to recognise a relapse because early treatment with steroids may help to speed recovery. However, steroids do not appear to improve the extent to which a person recovers from an attack and they can also have a lot of side effects. Treatment with steroids should therefore be kept to a minimum – they are not often given for mild

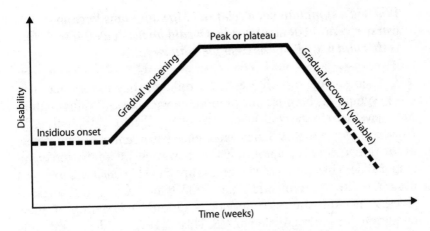

Figure 6.1 The time-course of a relapse in relapsing-remitting MS

relapses and are usually kept in reserve for more severe attacks. It is very important to avoid frequent and prolonged use of steroids because this increases the risk of developing diabetes, bone thinning (osteoporosis) and bone death (avascular necrosis), fractures, muscle wasting, stomach ulcers and infections.

It is also important to recognise what is not a true relapse (a so-called 'pseudo-relapse') in order to avoid unnecessary and inappropriate treatment with steroids. This can sometimes be quite difficult and there are no hard and fast rules. That said, if you develop new symptoms that have worsened over a few days or weeks, it is likely you are having a true relapse. However, if you develop a recurrence of old symptoms or a worsening of long-standing symptoms that last only a few hours in duration or wax and wane on a day-to-day basis, it is much more likely you are having a 'pseudo-relapse', particularly if it occurs at a time of an infection or stress.

If a person is having frequent and severe relapses, it is sensible to consider treatment to reduce the number and severity of attacks. This is known as *disease-modifying treatment* and includes drugs such as beta-interferon (Avonex, Betaferon, Extavia, Rebif 22/44), glatiramer acetate (Copaxone) and natalizumab (Tysabri) (see Chapter 8).

When is a symptom not a relapse?' My symptoms have got worse recently but my neurologist said it wasn't a relapse. Why is this and why didn't he treat me with steroids?

When someone with MS has a relapse, they experience new symptoms because one or more new patches of inflammation have developed in the central nervous system (brain and spinal cord). However, people with MS may experience a worsening of symptoms, or the return of old symptoms, without any new inflammation being responsible. These sorts of symptoms are called *'pseudo-relapses'* and are often due to an infection, particularly if there is an associated fever. A person may also develop a gradual worsening of their condition due to progression of MS. This sort of slow deterioration is not usually confused with a true relapse due to inflammation. That said, a slight deterioration due to progression (for example, a slightly increased clumsiness in a leg that is already weak and clumsy) may lead to a large increase in disability and be mistaken for a true relapse.

Steroids have been shown to speed up recovery from true relapses – those due to new inflammation – but are usually ineffective in situations where people are worse due to 'pseudo-relapses' or progression. Although steroids do seem to help some people who are not experiencing a true relapse, this is usually a temporary benefit. Steroids often give people a feeling of well-being for a short time and all drug treatments can have a positive placebo effect. Doctors do not usually like giving steroids unless there are significant new symptoms which suggest a troublesome relapse because of potential long-term side effects.

Are there any triggers which lead to a relapse, and what should I look out for?

A number of possible trigger factors have been studied over the years. It seems likely that viral infections may trigger a minority of relapses but the evidence to support a link with psychological stress is unconvincing. There is also no evidence for a link with physical trauma, including having an operation and a general anaesthetic. Reassuringly, there is also no evidence that vaccinations trigger relapses, and there is therefore no reason to avoid having them. Although it has been clearly established that the risk of having a relapse is increased for a few months following childbirth, this is counter-balanced by a reduced risk during pregnancy (see Chapter 19).

It is important to appreciate that so-called 'pseudo-relapses' may mimic true relapses and that these sorts of attacks tend to occur at times of infection or stress.

How can you tell if you're in remission? Do some symptoms lessen and disappear or do some stay for good?

The term 'remission' simply refers to the period of relative stability between relapses. In the early stages of relapsing-remitting MS, recovery from relapses is complete or substantial more than 80 per cent of the time and, as a consequence, a person may experience few or no symptoms during periods of remission. As time goes by and further relapses occur, a person may experience more symptoms during remission due to incomplete recovery from their relapses. These sorts of symptoms may be temporarily worsened or re-emerge at times of stress and infection – so-called 'pseudo-relapses'. Exercise and hot temperatures may also cause a brief re-emergence of symptoms previously experienced during a relapse – this is known as Uhthoff's phenomenon. For example, a person may experience blurred vision temporarily in one eye which was previously affected by optic neuritis. Unfortunately, it is not possible to predict the extent of recovery from a relapse or whether a person may experience a temporary recurrence or worsening of symptoms during periods of remission. If a person's condition starts to deteriorate slowly between relapses, this indicates that they have entered the progressive stage of the condition – secondary progressive MS.

Over what period of time do symptoms need to worsen to be called a relapse?

A relapse is usually defined as the development of new or recurrence of old neurological symptoms lasting at least 24 to 48 hours for which no other cause has been found. However, this definition tends to be used mainly for research purposes and it is not particularly helpful in routine clinical practice. In fact, most relapses are usually recognised by their nature and change with time. The types of symptoms typically experienced during relapses (as described at the beginning of this chapter) usually evolve over a few days, stabilise over a few weeks and then improve partially or completely over weeks to months.

It is important to recognise a relapse early in its evolution because treatment with steroids may speed recovery. Unfortunately, steroids do not appear to change the extent of recovery. It is also important to recognise what is not a true relapse – a so-called 'pseudo-relapse' – in order to avoid inappropriate steroid treatment and the associated side effects and risks. If in doubt, it is often useful to discuss your symptoms with your neurologist or MS nurse.

I recovered fully from my previous relapses but why have I not recovered as well this time?

R ecovery is usually substantial or complete in the majority of relapses that occur early in the course of relapsing-remitting MS. As a consequence, a person may experience few or no symptoms during periods of remission. Unfortunately, a person may experience more symptoms during remission over time due to incomplete recovery from subsequent relapses. This is due to the accumulation of injury caused to sensitive parts of the central nervous system from repeated attacks of inflammation.

Although it appears steroids speed recovery from relapses by reducing inflammation they do not appear to improve the extent of recovery. If you are experiencing frequent relapses with incomplete recovery, it may be relevant to consider treatment with disease-modifying drugs (see Chapter 8). These treatments reduce inflammation in the brain and spinal cord and, as a consequence, may reduce the number, and possibly the severity, of relapses. Unfortunately, the potential long-term benefit of these treatments in reducing the accumulation of disability over time is less certain.

How long will it take before I regain feeling in my lower limbs following a relapse?

A relapse causing loss of feeling in the lower limbs is usually due to a new area of inflammation in the spinal cord. This 'numbness' may sometimes be accompanied by weakness in the lower limbs, walking difficulties and bladder problems. Although it can be very difficult to predict how fully anyone might recover from a relapse, someone who has had a severe relapse may be less likely to make a speedy recovery. So a great deal of patience may be needed in following the advice provided by your neurologist, MS nurse and therapists.

If all types of relapse are considered, around 50 per cent (1 in 2) of people will have shown some improvement at 4 weeks, and around 70 per cent (7 in 10) by eight weeks. In people who do not make a complete early recovery, further more gradual improvement can continue for up to two years after a relapse.

I had a relapse three months ago in which I lost feeling in my arm. There hasn't been any improvement yet. How much longer must I wait before I know whether the feeling will come back?

If there has been little or no recovery after three months, full recovery is unlikely and many people will not notice much change from this time onward. Nevertheless, small and gradual improvements can sometimes occur for up to two years after a relapse. A lot of people find that even if there is little or no recovery, the problems they have will become less troublesome because they will adapt to them better and notice them less.

MANAGEMENT AND TREATMENT OF RELAPSES

I rang my MS nurse as I think I am having a relapse. All she suggested was that I rest. Why is this?

The management of a relapse depends upon several factors which include the duration and type of symptoms, their impact on your life and whether or not they have levelled off or are improving.

If your symptoms are mild, and perhaps if they relate to alteration or loss of sensation or they have only been present for a day or two, your MS nurse may advise you to rest, to conserve your energy and review the situation again in a day or two. It is important to eat regularly and get enough good quality sleep; sometimes symptoms can be more manageable as a result. If your symptoms continue to worsen despite these conservative measures and, in particular. if they are interfering with what you can do (in either your home or your work life) you should contact your MS nurse again. She will reassess your situation.

When and how should steroids be used?

Steroids should probably only be used in the treatment of relapses, and then only if the symptoms of a particular relapse are having a significant impact on that person's day-to-day activities. This is because steroids have significant side effects and risks. They are probably most effective when used early in the course of a relapse, when they are usually given in very high doses, typically over a few days.

The different sorts of steroids used include *prednisolone, methyl-prednisolone* and *dexamethasone*. Methylprednisolone is probably the most common steroid used. It is usually given in either in tablet form and via an infusion (drip in your arm) over 3 to 5 days. Occasionally, a lower reducing dose of steroids, or 'steroid tail' following on from the high dose course may be recommended. Prescribing steroids in tablet form has the advantage of expediency, whereas steroid infusions usually require hospital admission which may result in a delay in starting treatment.

Steroids are used to treat relapses because they often speed recovery. Surprisingly, the eventual recovery from a relapse is just as good if no steroids are given. This is one reason why steroids may not be recommended for what are considered to be mild relapses.

When should steroids not be used?

Steroids should not be used if the potential side effects and risks are considered to outweigh the potential benefits of treatment. Your neurologist, GP or MS nurse may not recommend steroids if the symptoms of a relapse are considered to be mild or if they have developed more than six weeks earlier. Neither are steroids likely to be recommended if your doctor believes you are having a 'pseudo-relapse' rather than a true relapse – if this occurs in the context of an infection, treatment with antibiotics may be more appropriate and steroids are best avoided. Steroids should not be used too frequently because the side effects and risks are probably linked to the total dose you receive over time. It is for this reason many doctors recommend no more than two courses of high dose steroids in any 12 month period, except in very unusual situations. If a person is having frequent significant relapses requiring repeated short courses of steroids, treatment with a disease-modifying drug may be more appropriate (see Chapter 8). Long-term continuous steroid treatment is not recommended.

I have completed a course of oral steroids. What should I feel like now they have stopped? They tasted awful!

It is not unusual to experience side effects during steroid treatment including poor sleep, mental agitation, euphoria and feeling flushed. Symptoms like this should begin to resolve once steroids have been stopped. You should start to notice an improvement in the symptoms of your relapse during treatment or shortly after it has finished. Unfortunately, the speed and the extent to which your symptoms may improve is impossible to predict on an individual basis.

I have heard that immunoglobulins can be used to treat relapses of MS. Is this true and what are they?

Immunoglobulins are *antibodies* that are produced by the body's immune system in response to a number of infective and non-infective triggers. The antibody and the trigger have a complementary shape so that they attach to each other like a key in a lock. Immunoglobulins are obtained from the samples of thousands of blood donors and are siphoned off (similar to petrol being refined from crude oil). Although blood donations are screened for a variety of infections such as HIV/AIDS, hepatitis B and C and syphilis, one cannot be certain that there is no risk of transmission of an infective agent from these products and this limits their widespread use. Also, because the availability of immunoglobulins depends upon blood donation, there are limited quantities. Immunoglobulins are required to treat other conditions and sometimes their use can be life-saving – for example, where people cannot produce their own antibodies.

Immunoglobulins can also be associated with side effects such as allergic reactions, non-infective meningitis and stroke. All of these factors mean they are rarely used in the UK to treat relapses of MS. However, there may be circumstances (for example, if you are unable for some reason to tolerate steroids) in which your neurologist may feel the use of immunoglobulins is justified. Trials of immuno-globulins in MS relapses have not been able to confirm their effectiveness, so they are unlikely to be used widely for this purpose.

7 | Principles of management in MS

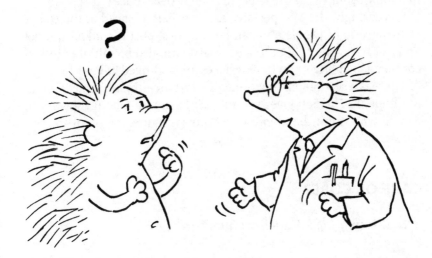

In general, there are three ways of managing MS: dealing with symptoms, managing acute relapses and modifying the course of the disease (the number and frequency of relapses and progression of disability over time). Symptom management and acute management of relapses have been considered in the two previous chapters, and more detailed information on symptoms and what to do about them is found later on in the book. This chapter looks at how we currently treat MS, while researchers are still striving to find a cure. We discuss our current understanding of the two compartment model of MS and the limitations of current treatments, before going on in the following chapter to look at disease-modifying treatments in more detail.

Now that I have been diagnosed with MS, who might I see?

The optimum management of MS requires a number of different health care professionals. You may not need to see all of them in the course of your illness, only those who are concerned with the treatment of the symptoms you are experiencing. Sometimes you may only require a single assessment, sometimes a course of treatment. Inevitably, your needs are likely to change over time.

Increasingly, the MS specialist nurse is being placed at the centre of this group of people and can be your first port of call for queries and referrals. Your GP and neurologist can also be initial points of contact depending upon how services are arranged in your locality.

There is a section on 'Relationships with healthcare professionals' in Chapter 22 which gives you more information about the various people who might be involved in your care at some point in your illness.

CARE OR CURE?

How is treating MS different from curing it?

A *cure* for MS would mean that after receiving it you would be completely healthy again as a result of the cure repairing the damage already caused to the brain and spinal cord and preventing any further damage occurring. A *treatment* seeks to reduce the impact of the disease by slowing or stopping the disease process. At present, we do not have a cure for MS and our treatments do not have the ability to regenerate damaged nerve cells. So, in practical terms, stopping the disease process is the next best outcome. In MS, our current treatments reduce inflammation and therefore relapses and short-term disability, and we hope this will slow down the rate of nerve cell death (neurodegeneration) which leads to long-term progression of disability. Treating people earlier in the course of MS, before they develop major disability, particularly with newer, more powerful anti-inflammatory drugs, may have a bigger impact on long-term disability. This may prove to the best option for managing people with MS in lieu of prevention or a cure.

If MS is not curable now, what does medical treatment achieve?

The treatment of MS consists of three strands; symptoms, relapses and disease modification (reduction in relapses and progression of disability). Medical treatment therefore seeks to:

- Reduce the impact of symptoms, such as pain, fatigue and spasticity;
- Reduce the length and severity of relapses with steroids;
- Improve the course of the condition with disease-modifying drugs.

Do you need to be on medication if you have MS?

Whether you need drug treatment will depend upon the symptoms you have, the relapses you experience and the availability of disease-modifying drugs that might potentially change the course of your type of MS.

Symptoms

You do not have to take drug treatment for MS. Whether or not you take a treatment for symptoms will depend upon the nature and the severity of the symptoms, how easy it is to take medication, potential side effects and risks. If you decide not to take a medication, you can always change your mind. If you are thinking of stopping or reducing a medication, it is important to discuss this first with your neurologist or MS nurse.

Relapses

Steroids are thought to accelerate the recovery you would have experienced without treatment. The decision whether or not to treat a relapse with steroids depends upon a number of factors. Firstly, the nature of your symptoms is important. If you are weak and/or your coordination is impaired, or if you are finding it difficult to walk, drive, work or fulfil your daily commitments to others, these are sound reasons why you and your neurologist and/or MS nurse may consider steroids are worthwhile. If you are a concert pianist, for example, changes in sensation in a hand would be very disabling as this would have a major impact on your earning power. But for most people, such a symptom might be irritating rather than incapacitating. The impact of symptoms on your life, therefore, should be talked through carefully with your MS nurse when you are discussing your management plan. However, if your symptoms have been present for some days or weeks, and are already spontaneously recovering, you may not get as much additional benefit from steroids as you would if you had taken them earlier in the course of the relapse. Again, discussing the advantages and disadvantages of steroids with your MS nurse will be helpful in this situation too.

More information about drug treatment of relapses can be found in Chapter 6.

Disease-modifying drugs

If you are eligible for treatment with a disease-modifying drug, whether or not you take one is a decision that is best made after discussion with your neurologist and MS specialist nurse. You should be given the opportunity to ask about the advantages and disadvantages of the treatment suggested, and talk through all the issues involved. Your decision should be an informed one, based upon the nature and likely course of your condition, potential benefits, side effects and risks.

The implications of not starting treatment should also be considered. It is often helpful to discuss these issues with close relatives or friends but it is important to try not to base your decision upon other people's experiences of a particular treatment. Everyone with MS is different and response to drug treatments can be difficult to predict.

More information about disease-modifying drugs can be found in Chapter 8.

THE TWO-STAGE MODEL

What is meant by the two-stage model of MS?

In people with relapsing-remitting MS, we know that early on in the course of their illness (the first stage) there is relatively more inflammation occurring within the brain and spinal cord. This can be demonstrated by the coming and going on MRI scans of white dots or plaques, and by the frequency of clinical attacks or relapses, which average around one every 12–18 months in the majority, but which can occur every few months in extreme cases. Although nerve cell death (neurodegeneration) does occur early on in MS, the majority of disability early on in the illness seems to be related to acute attacks of inflammation. As time passes, however, the amount of inflammation decreases, and consequently the number of new white dots or plaques and the number of relapses reduce. This is clearly seen year on year in studies where patients with MS received placebo (dummy) tablets. Even though they were not taking active medication, their relapses became less frequent in later years of the trials.

The number of relapses people experience in the early stages of their illness, and the degree of inflammation seen on MRI scans, seem less important than nerve cell death (which now predominates) in predicting the development of long-term disability. What does

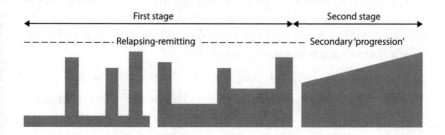

Figure 7.1 The two-stage model of MS

influence the course of MS critically is the development of slowly progressive disability due to nerve death (the second stage). Patients with an initial relapsing-remitting course tend, after a delay typically of several years, to worsen gradually over time. This is called secondary progressive MS. The majority of patients cease to relapse – or if they do, then they do so very infrequently.

This two-stage model of MS has been elegantly demonstrated by studies using a powerful anti-inflammatory drug called Campath 1H (now in Phase 3 clinical trials as *alemtuzumab*). If Campath is given to patients early on in the course of their disease, the results are almost a mirror image of those obtained when patients with secondary progressive MS are given the drug. In early MS, Campath almost completely stops relapses and also short-term progression of disability. In secondary progressive MS, where there is less inflammation, progressive disability appears to continue unaltered despite Campath. This led the research team to design a trial to test whether giving Campath (alemtuzumab) to patients within five years of the onset of their symptoms of MS, with recent evidence of MS activity (both relapses and new brain inflammation, white dots or plaques), was more effective in reducing relapses and sustained increases in disability, compared with what they considered to be the best standard disease-modifying drug (Rebif 44, three times weekly).

The results up to three years are impressive with Campath being over 70 per cent more effective than Rebif 44 in reducing relapse rates, sustained increases in disability and on a variety of MRI measures. Safety aspects of Campath are discussed in detail in the following chapter, but – as nerve cell death (neurodegeneration) seems to be the cause of long-term disability in MS – other fundamental questions remain to be answered:

- Is nerve cell death pre-programmed at some point in MS?

- If it is pre-programmed, when does this occur? (This will have big implications for when any treatments should be given.)

- Does inflammation cause long-term nerve cell death or are the two processes independent?

- Do any of our existing treatments prevent or delay nerve cell death, beyond question, in the long-term?

Perhaps the most interesting result from the Campath Phase 2 study will come from observing how these people with MS who have received potent anti-inflammatory treatment early in the course of their illness fare over the next few decades, and whether this intervention leads to stabilisation or slowing of their disability. In the meantime, the unanswered questions above introduce a number of issues which are discussed in the next two chapters on conventional and new disease-modifying treatments and research.

MONITORING PROGRESS

Is there any point in my continuing to see my consultant neurologist on a regular basis when it appears he can offer no further treatment?

Yes there is! Multiple sclerosis is a dynamic illness that is constantly evolving, and your condition will vary with time. Your needs may therefore change and a regular appointment with your neurologist or MS nurse will allow you to address any new queries. Developments in treatment, including results of clinical trials, are often reported in the media and it is important that you have the opportunity to discuss these if you wish. It is always worth reviewing your symptoms such as pain, bladder, spasticity and sleep quality from time to time to ensure that they are being treated adequately and to discuss whether you might benefit from additional drug treatment, change in medication or referral to a physiotherapist, occupational therapist, continence adviser or other allied health professional.

If either you or your neurologist does suggest discharge, it is important that you have easy access back into your local MS service. Usually, this can be achieved through contacting your MS specialist nurse, although your GP is another potential route.

I have been offered 'in-patient rehabilitation' in hospital. What will that mean?

It is likely that your neurologist, MS nurse or one of your therapists feels that you would benefit from an intensive and focused period of rehabilitation, preferably in a unit that specialises in this kind of care. A multidisciplinary team of doctor, physiotherapist, occupational therapist, psychologist and other members such as nutritionists and speech and language therapists will work with you to agree a series of graded steps or goals. The emphasis is very much on improving function and enabling you to maximise your potential and independence. You should expect to have a timetable of therapy and regular assessments of how you are progressing against your agreed goals. You should also expect to be an active member of this multidisciplinary team.

8 | Conventional disease-modifying drugs used in MS

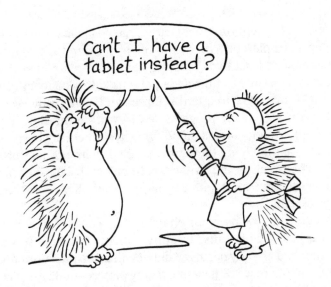

In this chapter we discuss issues relating to disease-modifying treatment for MS that are currently available for use in the UK (Avonex, Betaferon, Extavia, Rebif 22/44, glatiramer acetate (Copaxone) and natalizumab (Tysabri). Further information on them can be obtained from www.msdecisions.org.uk or from the websites of the MS Society and MS Trust (listed in Appendix 1). We go on to discuss the occasional use of other non-licensed disease-modifying drug treatments such as mitoxantrone (Novantrone) which your neurologist may consider in exceptional circumstances. Finally, we look at new developments in disease-modifying drugs, some of which are moving faster than others.

THE BENEFITS OF DISEASE-MODIFYING DRUGS

Can all patients with MS benefit from disease-modifying treatments?

In short, no. Current treatments are targeted against the treatment of relapses in patient with active relapsing-remitting MS, which usually means at least two clinically significant relapses within the previous 2 years. Only a minority of patients with secondary progressive MS will have very frequent relapses and, as a result, very few patients with secondary progressive MS will be thought likely to benefit from current disease-modifying treatments. There are no proven disease-modifying therapies for people with primary progressive MS. The precise criteria for treatment with beta-interferons, glatiramer acetate and natalizumab in the UK are outlined in Appendices 3 and 4.

As discussed in the previous chapter, the two-stage model theory of MS was proposed because treating patients in whom secondary progression had already occurred did not alter their accumulation of disability. Therefore we target our existing disease-modifying drugs in patients with relapsing-remitting MS earlier in their disease course, when relapses are more frequent, in the hope that this will improve the long-term prognosis. In addition, in patients with primary progressive MS, current disease-modifying treatments have failed to slow down or stop progression of disability.

If I am taking a disease-modifying drug, how will my neurologist evaluate whether it is working? Will she use scans or just go by what I put in my diary?

The short answer is that your neurologist will use all the information at her disposal to form an opinion about the efficacy of your treatment. The assessment that your neurologist will make to determine whether or not your disease-modifying drug is working will usually concentrate on whether you are having relapses less frequently now that you are on treatment, and on whether your degree of disability is stable. Disability may be measured by the Expanded Disability Status Scale (EDSS) for patients on the *Risk Sharing Scheme*. For other people, disability may be assessed by listening to their own assessment of how, for example, their walking has changed. A shortened version of the neurological examination may be carried out by a neurologist. A variety of other measures may be used which will vary from centre to centre. These may include the time it takes you to walk a distance (for example the 25 metre timed walk), measures of your cognitive faculties such as tests of concentration and memory including the Paced Auditory Serial Addition Test (PASAT), and the '9-hole peg test' which measures the time it takes you to place nine pegs in nine holes and remove them with each hand. If relapses are responsible for the increase in disability, there may be an option to change to an alternative disease-modifying treatment. If secondary progression is responsible for the increase in disability, currently there are no treatments that are proven to help slow down the worsening, and the neurologist may recommend stopping the treatment you are taking.

Some centres are now beginning to use MRI scans to reinforce the clinical impression about the effectiveness of particular treatments, but there is currently no overall agreement about whether, how often and how, this should be done.

If you are receiving treatment with beta-interferons (Avonex, Betaferon, Extavia, Rebif 22/44), you may have a blood test for *neutralising antibodies* or NABs. An antibody attaches to its complementary target, in this case the drug, like a key in a lock. This stops that molecule of the drug from exerting its effect and it is effectively like taking less of the drug. Sometimes, NABs may be checked routinely at certain intervals; in other centres some neurologists may only check them if the beta-interferon does not seem to be working very well. There is still controversy over the relevance of NABs, but there is beginning to be more consensus that persistent high levels appear to reduce the efficacy of beta-interferons.

Do disease-modifying drugs slow progression or treat symptoms?

If you are taking a disease-modifying drug, you should not expect it to decrease the number or severity of your *current* symptoms. Disease-modifying treatments are intended to prevent or delay relapses and symptoms in the future. In addition, all disease-modifying drugs have the potential to cause side effects in themselves. Around 10 per cent, or one in ten, people who take beta-interferons, for example, have to discontinue them because of side effects.

The rationale for prescribing a disease-modifying drug is that it reduces the inflammation in relapsing-remitting MS, as measured by reductions in new plaques on MRI scans, clinical relapses, and short-term accumulation of disability. It is this that causes a reduction in the development of new symptoms and, it is hoped, a slower progression of disability in the longer term. There is also evidence from trials that symptoms from new relapses may not be as severe in patients taking disease-modifying drugs as they are in those who do not.

How do I know that the disease-modifying drug my doctor has prescribed is the best one for me?

This is a difficult question! When your neurologist discussed the treatment options available to you, he or she may have already identified that some treatments may not have been appropriate for you. For example, the beta-interferons can trigger low mood and therefore doctors tend to avoid prescribing these in the first instance for people with a previous history of significant low mood. Your neurologist will have balanced the potential efficacy of the disease-modifying drug, given the activity of your MS and how it has developed over time, against the drug's tolerability profile and its potential for serious adverse effects. As a result, your neurologist may have offered you a choice of disease-modifying drugs, or directed you to a specific drug which he or she feels to be the best choice for you, based upon clinical knowledge and experience (including the results of clinical trials, seeing the treatment's effects in other patients with your MS type and course, and knowledge of your other medical conditions and personal circumstances including lifestyle).

It is not possible to predict the extent to which an individual drug will be effective for you. Therefore, it is important to note that taking the first choice drug does not necessarily rule out taking the other classes of drug in the future, but of course you are welcome to raise any concerns with your neurologist before you start treatment. Your neurologist will keep your response (or lack of response) to treatment under careful review and will offer alternative treatments if these appear to be indicated.

Whether you were offered a choice, or whether you were directed towards a particular treatment, it is important that you had enough information and time to be ready to commence treatment:

1 You have to be able to physically take your treatment via whichever route it is given. This can be difficult for the injectable treatments, the beta-interferons and glatiramer acetate, if you have weakness, reduced sensation or coordination in your hands and arms. Sometimes you may need someone to help you to take them.

2 You have to be able to tolerate any side effects of treatment. It is no use being unable to function in your daily life because the side effects of the treatments are too severe. Fortunately, this is not common.

3 You need to imagine that you will be taking the treatment for the foreseeable future and for at least as long as it still seems to be having a positive effect on the course of your MS and that there is no better alternative available.

If you can resolve these three issues then it will take at least several months and usually years before any positive effects of the disease-modifying drugs can be properly assessed. But you may notice a reduction in, or lack of, new symptoms, and a levelling out of any deterioration you had experienced before treatment. This may make you feel that the disease-modifying treatment you are taking is right for you before your neurologist necessarily confirms this.

If you are still in doubt about your treatment, you should discuss this with your neurologist or MS nurse.

Where can I find out more about the drugs that my GP has prescribed for me, and the side effects they may cause?

Every drug will have an information sheet inserted in its packaging. If this is not present, if you have lost it, or if you have any questions about the drug, you can either ask the pharmacist who dispensed it or the doctor or nurse who prescribed it. You can also find this information on the Internet. Appendix 1 includes some websites to help you with this.

If I stop disease-modifying drugs what will happen to me?

At present the available disease-modifying drugs reduce the number and rate of relapses by, on average, at least one third. We do not know conclusively that treatment with these agents has a marked effect on the progression of long-term disability.

The frequency of relapses in MS decreases year-on-year. This is clearly shown in those who receive placebo (dummy inactive treatment) in clinical trials of disease-modifying drugs. Therefore, to know whether stopping your medication makes a difference is likely to take some time. Some neurologists, if they were concerned about the activity of your MS, might wish you to have an MRI scan to look for evidence of a higher degree of activity, and may offer you an alternative disease-modifying treatment instead.

There is no clear evidence to suggest that people with relapsing-remitting MS who stop disease-modifying drugs have any rebound of their symptoms as a result of stopping treatment.

New trials of disease-modifying drugs in relapsing-remitting MS would be unethical if they did not offer the patient a chance of an active treatment which may have an effect at some stage in the trial.

Therefore, most new studies start by randomly allocating patients to an active drug or matching placebo dummy, without either the patient or the investigator knowing which treatment they are receiving. The patients are then followed up for a period of time, often around two years, and then all patients who satisfactorily complete the trial may then be offered the chance to take the active drug for a long-term extension study. As both the investigator and the patient know they are receiving the drug this is called open-label treatment. We now have two groups of patients; the 'Immediate' treatment group who have received the active drug from the start of the randomised trial and the 'Delayed' treatment group who initially received placebo. Although such long-term open-label trials are not ideal, as they tend to exaggerate any positive treatment effects, commonly there do appear to be small differences in outcomes favouring the 'Immediate' treatment group over those whose treatment was 'Delayed'. Whether or not these differences are big enough to be meaningful in the long-term is unknown but it may suggest that delaying treatment could be detrimental.

If you decline disease-modifying treatment when it is offered, but subsequently change your mind, it is possible that you may not then fulfil any treatment criteria at that stage. The simplest thing to do is to discuss this with your MS nurse or neurologist.

I gather that I could take beta-interferon if I had relapsing-remitting MS, but I have primary progressive MS. Are there any treatments for primary progressive MS?

Trials in progressive MS without relapses, that is primary progressive MS and non-relapsing secondary progressive MS, have been disappointing. Even very powerful treatments which reduce inflammation and have been proven to reduce relapses, have failed to show benefits in patients who have progression. This may relate to the dominant cause of progression of disability in primary progressive and non-relapsing secondary progressive MS being nerve cell death rather than inflammation (swelling).

Two recent studies, a large study of 900 patients using glatiramer acetate and another smaller trial using rituximab a monoclonal antibody, failed to show an overall effect in patients with primary progressive MS. However, it is possible that in primary progressive MS there may be differences in the amount of inflammation between younger patients with a shorter length of illness and these patients may be targeted for treatments in the future. Currently, however, the treatment of primary progressive MS is focused upon management of symptoms. You should not underestimate the positive impact upon your day-to-day quality of life of optimal management of symptoms such as pain, bladder and spasticity management. If nothing else, this can improve your sleep which will, in turn, help to minimise the effects of fatigue.

I recently heard about beta-interferon and how it could help MS, so I went to my GP to ask for it. She said she could not prescribe it. Why?

In the UK, prescription of certain disease-modifying drugs for MS such as beta-interferon (Avonex, Betaferon, Extavia, Rebif 22/44), glatiramer acetate (Copaxone) and natalizumab (Tysabri) is limited to neurologists with expertise in the management of people with MS. This arrangement helps to ensure access to these expensive treatments is equitable and that people started on these drugs are assessed and monitored appropriately.

Lots of people I know are now talking about beta-interferons, as a way of controlling MS. It sounds almost like a cure to me. Is it?

No. There are four beta-interferons available for the treatment of MS: Avonex, Betaferon, Extavia and Rebif 22/44. Interferons are produced naturally in the body and help cells communicate with each other. The three beta-interferon drugs have slightly different properties, frequencies and routes of administration but, on average, reduce one in three relapses and short-term disability over a few years. Their effects on the development of irreversible long-term disability is less certain as long-term placebo controlled trials have never been conducted, and probably now never will be. Most neurologists would agree that although they have an undoubted treatment effect in MS, beta-interferons are, at best, partially effective. Some patients do remain relatively stable, whereas others continue to relapse and convert to secondary progressive MS with increasing disability over time and therefore the beta-interferons do not represent a cure for MS.

Can disease-modifying drugs like beta-interferons and glatiramer acetate help everyone with MS?

No – it is important to note that not all patients with MS will have sufficiently frequent relapses to benefit clearly from these drugs. The major studies which tested the effectiveness of beta-interferon and glatiramer acetate in MS examined only a proportion of people with relapsing-remitting MS. They took patients with relapsing-remitting MS and above average relapse rates of at least two relapses within the previous two years (or at least one relapse in the previous year with glatiramer acetate). These patients were still able to walk at least 100 metres without stopping, aid or assistance. In these patients, beta-interferon or glatiramer acetate reduced the relapse rate by about 30 per cent in addition to the reduction seen in patients on placebo dummy medication. Only one of four studies of beta-interferons in people with secondary progressive MS showed a benefit; this is thought to be due to the fact that in this study patients had more relapses contributing to their disability. Beta-interferons had no effect on disability progression in patients with secondary progressive MS without relapses. Both beta-interferons and glatiramer acetate have failed to show a benefit in reducing disability rates in people with primary progressive MS.

Does beta-interferon, or any other drug, delay the development of disability in MS?

In order to answer this question it is necessary to do clinical trials that compare an active drug to a placebo ('dummy drug'). It is also necessary for such trials to run for many years in order to be confident any beneficial effect a drug may have on disability is sustained and big enough to be clinically meaningful. Unfortunately, the vast majority of clinical trials of disease-modifying drugs run for only a few years, and therefore the long-term effects these treatments may have on disability are uncertain. However, it is possible to gain some insights by looking at the clinical trial results of these drugs in the earlier and later stages of MS.

Clinical trials of beta-interferons (Avonex, Betaferon, Rebif 22/44), glatiramer acetate (Copaxone), and more aggressive treatments including mitoxantrone (Novantrone), natalizumab (Tysabri) and alemtuzumab (Campath) in relapsing-remitting MS have generally shown that people receiving the active drug are less disabled than those on placebo ('dummy drug'). The beneficial effects are generally bigger for the stronger drugs like natalizumab (Tysabri) and alemtuzumab (Campath), but at the cost of significantly higher risks of serious adverse effects. This may sound encouraging for a beneficial effect of drug treatment on long-term disability. However, much of the effect on disability measurements in these clinical trials in relapsing-remitting MS may be due to a reduction in the number of relapses rather than a reduction in disease progression itself. This notion is supported by the lack of any convincing effect on disability when these very same drugs are trialled in people with primary and secondary progressive MS.

Long-term studies, which would tell us whether drugs like beta-interferon reduce the chances of people with relapsing-remitting MS converting to secondary progressive MS, are difficult to do. This is because once a drug has been shown to have some benefits (such as reduction in relapse rate) the clinical trial is stopped on ethical grounds and the active drug is then offered to the people who were initially receiving placebo ('dummy drug'). As a consequence, it is not known whether early treatment with beta-interferon, or any other drugs, influences long-term prognosis. That said, these drugs are generally used in the earlier stages of MS in the hope that they will have a long-term beneficial effect on disability.

How do you take beta-interferon? I've heard that you need injections, and I hate jabs!

You are right to say that the four beta-interferons (Avonex, Betaferon, Extavia, Rebif 22/44) and glatiramer acetate (Copaxone) are all given as injections (see Table 8.1). Unfortunately, these drugs do not work when given in tablet form. Your MS nurse should demonstrate how to give yourself the injection safely and efficiently, and teach you ways of reducing side effects such as discomfort.

I have been offered a choice of four injectable disease-modifying drugs (three beta-interferons and glatiramer acetate). What are the differences between them?

In terms of reducing relapse rates and preventing long-term disability, no large study comparing all four drugs simultaneously, has been undertaken for a long enough time to detect any statistically significant and clinically meaningful difference in treatment effect.

Where these drugs do differ is in their method of manufacture, the route and frequency of administration, whether or not the drug needs to be made into a liquid from its original powdered form and how it must be stored (see Table 8.1). All these drugs also differ in their side effect profile and the three beta-interferons differ in their tendency to cause *neutralising antibodies* (NABs). Unfortunately, all these drugs are potentially teratogenic (harmful to the baby in the event of pregnancy) and it is therefore important to take contraceptive precautions and stop treatment in advance if you are intending to get pregnant.

Table 8.1 summarises these differences and may help you choose the right drug for you. Occasionally there are changes to these

Table 8.1 Characteristics of beta-interferons and glatiramer acetate

Drug	Method of manufacture	Excipients	Dose	Rate of administration
Avonex	Produced in Chinese hamster ovary cells by DNA technology	Human serum albumin, Dibasic sodium phosphate, Monobasic sodium phosphate, Sodium chloride	30 μg	IM
Betaferon Extavia**	Produced by genetic engineering from strain of bacteria *Escherichia coli*	Human albumin Mannitol Sodium chloride Water for injection	250 μg	SC
Rebif	Produced in Chinese hamster ovary cells by recombinant DNA technology	Mannitol Poloxamer 188 L methionine Benzyl alcohol Sodium acetate Acetic acid Sodium hydroxide Water for injections	22 μg or 44 μg	SC
Glatiramer acetate	Acetate salt of synthetic polypeptides, containing four naturally occurring amino acids: L-glutamic acid, L-alanine, L-tyrosine and L-lysine	Mannitol Water for Injections	20 mg	SC

*NABs = Neutralising Antibodies; IM = Intramuscular; SC = Subcutaneous

uency min- tion	Storage	Need to reconstitute powdered drug before injecting	Administration time following reconstitution	Rate of NABs* for formation
e weekly	Less than 25°C Do not freeze	Yes	Should be administered as soon as possible after reconstitution but can be stored at 2°C to 8°C for up to six hours, prior to injection. Bring it out half an hour before injecting	2–5%
rnate days	Less than 25°C Do not freeze	Yes	After reconstitution an immediate use is recommended but stability has been demonstrated for 3 hours at 2–8 °C	up to 45%
ee times ekly	Store in a refrigerator (2°C to 8°C) Do not freeze. Store in the original package in order to protect from light	No	Not applicable	12.5–24%
ily	Store in a refrigerator (2°C to 8°C). If the pre-filled syringes cannot be stored in a refrigerator, they can be stored at room temperature (15°C to 25°C), once for up to one month, but if unused must be returned to a refrigerator	No	Keep the container in the outer carton, in order to protect from light	Not applicable

Extavia and Betaferon are identical drugs with different brand names. They differ only in their injection apparatus and support services parameters and you should check with your neurologist and MS nurse for up-to-date information about these products. Details of how to access more up-to-date information online can be found in Appendix 1.

I have been offered a new drug called Extavia. What is this?

Extavia is a branded version of beta-interferon 1b, which is identical to the drug Betaferon. Extavia was launched in the UK in April 2009. Where the two brands differ is in the apparatus used to inject them. Your MS nurse or neurologist will be able to explain these and any other minor differences.

I'm currently being treated with a beta-interferon. My doctor wants to do a blood test for neutralising antibodies – why?

All four of the beta-interferons (Avonex, Betaferon, Extavia, Rebif 22/44) are associated with the development of neutralising antibodies. They usually develop within the first few years of treatment and they may sometimes disappear over time. Betaferon and Extavia are the drugs most likely to cause neutralising antibodies whereas Avonex is the least likely and Rebif 22/44 is somewhere in between.

Although neutralising antibodies do not cause symptoms and are not harmful in themselves, there is evidence to indicate they reduce the effectiveness of treatment. Unfortunately, there is currently no consensus between neurologists as to how they should be dealt with. In 2005, a body of experts (European Federation of Neurological Societies Task Force) recommended routine testing at one and two years from the start of treatment. The same body recommended that treatment should be stopped in anyone with persistently high levels. In 2007, a second body of experts (Therapeutics and Technology Assessment Subcommittee of the American Academy of Neurology) accepted that sustained high levels of neutralising antibodies reduced the effectiveness of treatment but that there was insufficient information to recommend when to test, which test to use and how many tests are necessary. In the same year, a third body of experts (Association of British Neurologists) recommended that neutralising antibody test results should be used to support a decision to stop treatment only if there is concern it is not working because of continuing relapses or MRI evidence of disease activity.

Neutralising antibodies can be detected with a blood test. Your neurologist should be able to explain why you need to be tested and what is likely to be recommended if the test is positive – you may be advised to stop treatment or switch to a different disease-modifying drug.

You have talked a lot about the beta-interferon drugs, but my friend was given steroid drugs when she had an attack of MS. What are steroid drugs?

Steroids are potent substances which are made naturally by your body and can be given by your doctor as tablets or via an infusion (a 'drip'). They have a whole variety of beneficial and potentially harmful effects.

Steroids reduce inflammation and can therefore accelerate the recovery you would have made from your relapse, but they don't have additional beneficial effects. They tend to be most effective early in the course of relapsing-remitting MS and some patients notice the beneficial effect of each successive course of steroids is less impressive than the last. It has not been established beyond doubt whether high dose steroids given in tablet form (usually of methylprednisolone, sometimes prednisolone or dexamethasone) or via an infusion ('a drip' – usually methylprednisolone) are any different in terms of their positive effects. Some neurologists also give a reducing course of steroids (with the dose tapering down) for a week or longer if your relapse has been particularly bad.

Steroids have a number of potential side effects. In the short term they can have effects on mood including making you feel up or down. They can also make your mind race and your face blush. If steroids are given too frequently (for example more than twice a year) there is an increased risk of more serious long-term effects. These include interruption of the blood supply to the hip bone (avascular necrosis of the femoral head). This effectively causes a 'stroke' of the bone and, as a consequence, the worst case scenario would involve a hip replacement. If you develop any difficulties walking or hip pain following a course of steroids, you should discuss this with your neurologist or MS nurse. When steroids are used frequently or on a long-term basis, they can also cause weight gain, high blood pressure, diabetes and osteoporosis (bone thinning). It is therefore very important to keep steroid use to a minimum and avoid continuous treatment. If you are having frequent relapses it is important to consider whether starting a disease-modifying drug is a more sensible treatment option.

I have progressive MS. My doctor says that neither disease-modifying drugs nor steroids are going to help me. Is that really the case?

At present none of the currently used disease-modifying drugs have been shown to be effective in patients with progressive forms of MS. This may be due to the fact that people with primary and secondary progressive MS have relatively little inflammation compared to those with relapsing-remitting MS and that disability appears to be related predominantly to nerve cell death (neurodegeneration). If you have never had steroids and the type of MS you have is unclear, your neurologist may discuss with you whether a single course of high dose steroids is indicated in the rare event they may be helpful. Careful monitoring for any sustained and meaningful response would need to be undertaken to avoid the risks of further unnecessary courses of steroids where there has been no objective effect.

Is it safe to combine drugs like steroids with disease-modifying drugs like beta-interferon (Avonex, Betaferon, Rebif 22/44), glatiramer acetate (Copaxone) and natalizumab (Tysabri)?

There are not thought to be specific problems with taking steroids with any of these medications at the same time if, for example, you have a relapse which requires treatment. At present there is, however, no convincing evidence that taking steroids *regularly* together with one of the other disease-modifying drugs leads to additional reductions in relapse rates.

Whether it is safe to take more than one disease-modifying drug together is a more difficult question to answer. Two cases of a virally triggered brain disorder called *progressive multifocal leucoencephalopathy (PML)* occurred in patients taking Avonex and natalizumab (Tysabri) together. Generally, therefore, combination treatment with more than one disease-modifying drug at a time is neither offered nor recommended. At the time of writing, there is an ongoing clinical trial with Avonex and glatiramer acetate examining the safety and efficacy of this drug combination. Some neurologists in the UK use mitoxantrone (Novantrone) and overlap its use with glatiramer acetate. Mitoxantrone, however, is currently unlicensed in the UK. See below for more information on licensed and unlicensed drugs.

It sounds from what you have said about the promise of the new disease-modifying drugs that I hardly need to worry about other ways of managing my MS. Is that so?

No! Disease-modifying drugs should not be considered to be a panacea for all ills in MS. They should not be expected to have an effect on your immediate day-to-day symptoms but be considered as a preventative measure to reduce the impact of your condition on your life over future years. Therefore, whether you are taking disease-modifying drugs or not, you should still pay attention to the appropriate and timely treatment of symptoms and relapses together with general lifestyle changes such as healthy living, exercise and diet.

SIDE EFFECTS

I have heard that the injectable disease-modifying therapies have lots of side effects – is this true?

The five disease-modifying therapies given by injection are Interferon beta 1a (Avonex and Rebif); interferon beta 1b (Betaferon and Extavia) and glatiramer acetate (Copaxone). Four of these are administered subcutaneously (just under the skin), whereas Avonex is injected into a muscle once a week.

Each of these medications can cause side effects (as can any medication) though there is a great deal that can be done to minimise any problems you may have. Your MS nurse will talk this through with you when you start. Starting Rebif and Betaferon or Extavia at lower doses and gradually increasing the dose can help to minimise side effects (see Tables 8.2 and 8.3).

Table 8.2 Betaferon and Extavia

Patients should be started at 62.5 µg (0.25 ml) subcutaneously every other day, and increased slowly to a dose of 250 µg (1.0 ml) every other day. The titration period may be adjusted, if any significant adverse reaction occurs. In order to obtain adequate efficacy, a dose of 250 µg (1.0 ml) every other day should be reached.

Schedule for dose titration*

Treatment day	Dose	Volume
1, 3, 5	62.5 µg	0.25 ml
7, 9, 11	125 µg	0.5 ml
13, 15, 17	187.5 µg	0.75 ml
19 and beyond	250 µg	1.0 ml

*The titration period may be adjusted, if any significant adverse reaction occurs.

Table 8.3 Rebif

The Rebif initiation pack allow patients to begin treatment of 8.8 µg for 2 weeks, then 22 µg for 2 weeks. Some patients will then begin on 44 µg.

Schedule for dose titration

Treatment week	Dose
1, 2	8.8 µg
3, 4	22 µg
5 and beyond	44 µg*

* If tolerated

The side effects that people are most likely to experience are either injection site reactions or a systemic effect a couple of hours after the injection and these are dealt with in the two questions below.

My friend has just started to inject herself with one of the disease-modifying therapies and is having a lot of problems at the injection sites – is this common?

Betaferon, Extavia, Copaxone and Rebif can all result in injection site reactions (because Avonex is injected into a muscle it tends to cause fewer problems at the injection site though people may still experience bruising or a little bleeding at times). Common reactions may include a raised reddened area, bruising, itching, pain and lumpiness. Often, people just experience a red mark at the injection site – a little like a thumb print – which fades in time. Copaxone may also cause dips in the skin at the injection site (lipoatrophy), though not everyone experiences this.

There is much that can be done to alleviate any problems people may experience at their injection sites. When your friend started on her treatment, she would have received training in how best to give the injections and how to manage the potential side effects. The MS nurse would have demonstrated how to give the injection both manually and using a pen-like device (often called an auto-injector) specific to the medication she is using.

Good injection technique makes a big difference in helping to minimise any injection site reactions, and rotation of the injection sites is particularly important. The MS nurse will have shown your friend the eight different areas to use; diagrams, instruction booklets and DVDs are provided with each of the different treatments for your friend to refer back to if needs be. Some people do find that some sites are more tender than others. These areas can be avoided for a little while, although it is important to rotate around as many of the different sites as possible to give the skin the maximum amount of time to heal between injections.

Other tips which can help minimise any pain your friend may be experiencing when she injects include making sure the injection is at room temperature before injecting, and injecting with a dry needle – if a droplet of the medication is present on the end of the needle then a gentle shake or tap can help. Some people also find that either gently cooling or warming the skin prior to injecting can help.

If your friend is experiencing pain, redness, itching or inflammation at the injection sites, she may find an anti-inflammatory cream (such as arnica) is helpful. Other people find an antihistamine cream, or a mild hydrocortisone cream, may help with more persistent problems. If your friend is not sure what may help, she should contact her MS nurse who will be very experienced in dealing with this sort of problem and will be able to give more specific advice.

It is important to remember that even though some people do experience side effects from these medications, there is much that can be done to help. Also, the benefits of the medications generally out-weigh any other problems they may cause. The MS nurse is there to give advice and support to anyone using these medications.

I am due to go for assessment soon, to see whether I am suitable for one of the disease-modifying therapies. But I am worried about the potential side effects. I have heard that they can make you feel ill – is this the case?

All five of the injectable disease-modifying therapies discussed above can cause some side effects that can make you feel off colour for a while, though for the vast majority of people this is no more than a minor and passing inconvenience.

The four interferon beta injections (Avonex, Betaferon, Extavia and Rebif) all have similar side effects in that they can make you feel a bit fluey for a few hours after each injection. This may be experienced as just feeling a bit more tired and achy than usual, or as more like 'flu with shivering and generally feeling poorly (though this is unusual). When you start on treatment your MS nurse will talk to you about all the potential side effects and how to manage them. People are usually advised to take their injections at night before going to bed and to take a couple of paracetamol or ibuprofen with them. This way most people are able to sleep through the 'flu-like symptoms and the paracetamol or ibuprofen mitigates the worst of the symptoms. It is important to bear in mind that these symptoms wear off after a few weeks (or even earlier) anyway. If you do continue to have problems with these symptoms then discuss them with your MS nurse.

Glatiramer acetate (Copaxone) has a different side effect profile. People taking Copaxone don't get 'flu-like symptoms and often don't get any systemic effects at all. However, some people do experience a post-injection reaction which typically comes on within 30 minutes of the injection being given. The individual feels as though their heart is racing, their chest is tight, it may feel difficult to breathe and can be very scary. This typically only lasts a few minutes and then resolves as quickly as it started. It is important to remember that this reaction has been exhaustively investigated and that, while it may feel quite uncomfortable at the time, it is quite benign and will not cause any harm. Many people will never experience this, those who do will typically be troubled only once or twice a year. Your MS nurse will discuss all this with you before you start treatment.

What about the side effects of new disease-modifying drugs? Don't all powerful drugs have side effects?

It is becoming clearer that as new, more powerful, disease-modifying drugs for MS are becoming available, there is a trade-off with an increased risk of more significant side effects. Any new drug may be teratogenic (harmful to the baby in the event of pregnancy) and this potential risk is unknown. Your neurologist should discuss the disease-modifying drugs they think are suitable for you and explain the potential side effects and risks of these treatments. Your neurologist should also inform you if there is any increase in known side effects or new risks over time, once you have started treatment. If you are concerned and you are not in regular contact with your neurologist or MS nurse you may wish to contact them either directly or via your GP.

IMMUNOSUPPRESSIVE DRUGS

I've heard about immunosuppressive treatments – what are they and do they have a role in the treatment of MS?

As their name suggests, these sorts of treatments suppress the immune system. Most of them have been in widespread use for many years and they are usually used to treat conditions caused by a malfunctioning immune system. Unfortunately, they all have significant side effects, require regular blood test monitoring and have significant risks including infections, cancer and reduced fertility. They are all potentially teratogenic (harmful to the baby in the event of pregnancy) and it is therefore important to take contraceptive precautions and stop treatment if you are intending to get pregnant.

A number of immunosuppressive drugs have been investigated as potential treatments for MS. However, most of the major clinical trials were performed a number of years ago and they have tended to be much smaller and less well designed than those of the newer immunomodulatory treatments such as beta-interferon (Avonex, Betaferon, Extavia, Rebif 22/44) and glatiramer acetate (Copaxone). As a consequence, the evidence is usually less robust, sometimes inconclusive and occasionally contradictory. In view of all these considerations, immunosuppressive treatments are not used routinely but may have an important role in certain situations. The sorts of immunosuppressive drugs sometimes used in MS include azathioprine, cyclophosphamide and mitoxantrone (Novantrone). Autologous haematopoeitic stem cell transplantation is another form of immunosuppressive treatment.

Azathioprine
Azathioprine is probably the most widely used immunosuppressive drug in MS. It is given as a tablet once a day. Clinical trials have shown it may have similar benefits to beta-interferon (Avonex, Betaferon, Extavia, Rebif 22/44) and glatiramer acetate (Copaxone) but this is uncertain because there have been no direct head-to-head comparisons. Unfortunately, it can often cause troublesome side effects including nausea, vomiting and diarrhoea and requires regular blood test monitoring. A test for an enzyme called TPMT can indicate whether it is safe to start treatment and at what dose. There is also a potential long-term risk of cancer that may be dose-related. Nevertheless, it may be considered to be a reasonable alternative to beta-interferon (Avonex, Betaferon, Extavia, Rebif 22/44) and glatiramer acetate (Copaxone) in certain situations.

Cyclophosphamide
Cyclophosphamide is a powerful immunosuppressive drug used in a variety of conditions, but its use in MS is controversial. It is usually given via intravenous infusion ('a drip') every few weeks but can be given in tablet form. It has significant side effects including nausea,

vomiting and hair loss and the total dose that can be given is usually limited due the risk of cancer. Unfortunately, the results of early clinical trials were contradictory and its routine use in MS cannot therefore be recommended. However, the results of more recent clinical trials indicate it may have a role in the treatment of people with rapidly worsening MS, providing the benefits are considered to outweigh the risks. That said, other powerful immunosuppressive drugs such as mitoxantrone (Novantrone) may be considered in this specific situation, as could new immunomodulatory treatments like natalizumab (Tysabri).

Mitoxantrone

Mitoxantrone (Novantrone) is another powerful immunosuppressive drug given via intravenous infusion ('a drip'). It is generally better tolerated than cyclophosphamide but it has similar risks including infection, cancer and reduced fertility. Unfortunately, it can only be used on a short-term basis because of the risk of heart problems (cardiotoxicity). Clinical trials have shown it can reduce relapse rate by over two-thirds and it is therefore likely to be more effective than beta-interferon (Avonex, Betaferon, Extavia, Rebif 22/44) and glatiramer acetate (Copaxone). It is a reasonable treatment option for people with rapidly worsening MS, as long as the significant risks are borne in mind. If mitoxantrone appears to beneficial, a switch to an immunomodulatory drug such as a beta-interferon (Avonex, Betaferon, Extavia, Rebif 22/44) or glatiramer acetate (Copaxone) may be considered.

Stem cell transplantation

Autologous haematopoeitic stem cell transplantation is probably the most aggressive form of immunosuppression used in MS. Its use is very controversial. This form of treatment requires the collection of stem cells from blood followed by destruction of the person's immune system with chemotherapy, and then replacement of the stem cells. Initial studies showed this treatment had a mortality (death) rate of 10 per cent (1 in 10) although this may now be lower with more careful patient selection. Its routine use is not recommended outside of clinical trials.

NON-LICENSED DISEASE-MODIFYING DRUG TREATMENTS

What do you mean by a licensed drug?

There are a number of steps required to prove the efficacy and safety of a drug before a regulatory authority will grant a licence for it to be used in a particular condition. Firstly, the drug is tested in a small number of healthy volunteers for safety (Phase 1 study). Secondly, a larger trial is undertaken (Phase 2 study) with people with the particular condition in order to determine the dose range and safety profile of the drug, usually together with a measure of treatment efficacy. For a disease-modifying drug in MS, the efficacy outcome in Phase 2 studies is usually based upon changes on MRI scans rather than clinical measures such as relapses and disability. Finally, if a Phase 2 study shows promise, a much larger Phase 3 study with several hundred people is conducted. For a disease-modifying drug in MS, the primary outcome measure is usually a change in the number of relapses or disability compared with another disease-modifying drug or placebo ('dummy drug'). The pharmaceutical company will then present all of its efficacy and safety data on the drug to the regulatory authority, who will then consider granting a licence for its use. It is not unusual for a regulatory authority to require a second Phase 3 study to be performed before a licence is granted and it is now commonplace for Phase 4 studies to be conducted once a drug gains a licence in order that the safety profile of the drug can continue to be monitored. More information about drug trials can be found in Chapters 9 and 10.

Some licensed drugs are prescribed 'off licence' – that is, they are given for a condition or symptom for which the drug was not originally granted a licence. For example, your neurologist may recommend treatment with amitriptyline – a tricyclic antidepressant – for nerve (neuropathic) pain because there is a body of anecdotal evidence that it may be beneficial (unlicensed indication). Your neurologist should talk to you about this, as well as explaining about its potential benefits, side effects and risks.

I have heard that an anti-cancer drug called mitoxantrone can help some patients with MS. What is this?

Mitoxantrone (Novantrone) is a drug which was developed to treat certain types of cancer (chemotherapy). It works in MS by reducing the number of T-cells (lymphocytes). There have been a number of clinical trials which have investigated the use of mitoxantrone in people with various types of MS. It appears to work best in people with frequent relapses or in those who develop rapid worsening of disability in a short period of time. It is given via an intravenous infusion ('a drip') at monthly to three monthly intervals. In common with other chemotherapy drugs, to avoid it being given by mistake to another person, it is deliberately dyed a blue colour and will stain your urine.

Unfortunately, the total amount of mitoxantrone, and therefore the duration of treatment that can be given, is limited because of the risk of damage to the heart (cardiotoxicity). This side effect is much more likely to occur at higher total doses. The risk increases with total dose used and therefore modern regimens use as little mitoxantrone as possible. When mitoxantrone is used carefully in this way, the risk of cardiotoxicity is likely to be less than 1 in 200 treated patient (0.5%). Mitoxantrone can also cause cancer of the blood cells (leukaemia) which is potentially fatal. This risk of developing this complication is harder to predict as it is not as clearly related to the total dose given and usually occurs in about 0.25 per cent (1 in 400) of people treated. Other side effects include thinning of hair although usually not total loss like other chemotherapy drugs, an increased risk of infections for a few weeks after each dose and disturbed menstrual periods with the possibility of an early menopause, particularly in women over 35. It is potentially teratogenic (harmful to the baby in the event of pregnancy) and it is therefore important to take contraceptive precautions and stop treatment well in advance if you are intending to get pregnant.

Mitoxantrone is only licensed for use in certain types of cancer. If your neurologist is considering treating you with it (unlicensed indication), a careful discussion of its potential benefits, side effects and risks will need to take place and the option of alternative licensed treatments considered. As the duration of treatment with mitox-antrone is limited, some neurologists follow treatment with other disease-modifying drugs such as beta-interferon (Avonex, Betaferon, Extavia, Rebif 22/44) or glatiramer acetate (Copaxone).

What about intravenous immunoglobulin – does it work in MS?

Intravenous immunoglobulin (IVIG) is obtained from the blood donations of thousands of healthy people. It is a licensed treatment used in a wide variety of different conditions unrelated to MS. A Phase 3 clinical trial of intravenous immunoglobulin in relapsing-remitting MS showed it reduced relapse rate by about a third – a benefit similar to that identified with beta-interferon (Avonex, Betaferon, Extavia, Rebif 22/44) and glatiramer acetate (Copaxone). Unfortunately, it was not shown to be of any benefit in the treatment of people with secondary progressive MS. It is usually given via intravenous infusion ('a drip') every few weeks and is generally well tolerated. All potential donors have to be screened for blood-borne infections including hepatitis viruses and HIV as a precaution – even so, there is always concern about the possibility of contamination by some unidentifiable infectious agent. Intravenous immunoglobulin appears to be a reasonable treatment option in people with relapsing-remitting MS. However, it is not routinely used because it is not licensed for use in MS, supplies are very limited and other disease-modifying drugs are available.

9 | New disease-modifying treatments used in MS

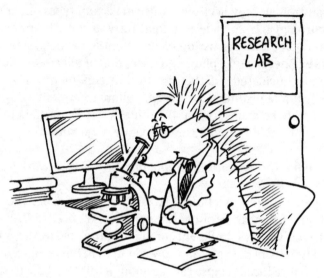

All drugs have to go through a lengthy period of development and testing before they can be licensed for use on patients. This chapter looks at some disease-modifying drugs which are not yet licensed because they are still at this development stage, though in a year or two that might have changed. In the meantime, you are likely to hear about some of them and you may even be participating in a trial involving one of them (more information about clinical trials is given in Chapter 10).

What promising disease-modifying treatments are on the horizon for MS?

There are always a number of drugs in development for MS and listing them all would not allow one to 'see the wood for the trees'. We have not listed treatments which may be used in combination.

Rather, we have divided promising single new treatments into three sections; monoclonal antibodies, oral treatments (tablets) and 'other'. In order to be listed here a potential treatment must have be shown to be 'broadly safe' (Phase 1 study data) and have shown early promise in a trial of people with MS (Phase 2 study data). This does *not* mean that there is absolutely no risk of potentially life-threatening side effects. Demonstration of safety is an *ongoing* process which continues into Phase 3 and 4 studies, and in clinical practice after a drug has been licensed for use.

Usually, this means that the drug has shown a significant reduction compared with placebo (dummy drug) in some form of outcome on MRI imaging. Sometimes this is reduction in the number of new plaques or the total number of plaques. Drugs like this, that have shown promise in Phase 2 studies, are likely to be undergoing Phase 3 trials or may be soon, where their effect on reduction in relapses and short-term disability will be examined. Providing they demonstrate benefit and safety in Phase 3 trials, these drugs may be available for prescription in the future.

It should be emphasised that you cannot directly compare the trial results of the agents we discuss in this chapter. The reason for this is that the studies did not have the same inclusion and exclusion criteria, that is the characteristics of the groups of people with MS in each trial were not the same. Unless otherwise stated, the following drugs are potential new treatments for people with relapsing-remitting MS only at the current time.

The table below gives some outline information about these drugs for your reference. You should be aware that the order in which these drugs are listed in their broad classes is for illustration only. The estimated dates of completion for the pivotal Phase 3 studies are subject to change, and there will be other issues that need to be resolved before any drug may or may not receive a licence for use in MS.

Nevertheless this list is not meant to be exhaustive and will date quickly. Therefore, the reader is advised to look at the websites of the MS Society, the MS Trust or other relevant websites listed in Appendix 1 for up-to-date information.

Table 9.1 Potential new disease-modifying drugs for MS

Class	Drug [company]	Estimated finish date of pivotal Phase 3 trial (name) or results
Oral (tablet)	Cladribine [Merck Serono]	Completed (CLARITY) 50% reduction in relapse rate compared with placebo
Oral (tablet)	Fingolimod/FTY720 [Novartis]	July 2009 (FREEDOMS)
Oral (tablet)	Teriflunomide [Sanofi Avensis]	October 2010 (TEMSO)
Oral (tablet)	Laquinimod [Teva Neuroscience]	March 2011 (ALLEGRO)
Oral (tablet)	BG00012/Fumarate [Biogen Idec]	December 2010 (DEFINE) April 2011 (CONFIRM)
Monoclonal antibody	Alemtuzumab (Campath) [Genzyme/Bayer Schering]	March 2011 (CARE MS-1) April 2012 (CARE MS-2)
Monoclonal antibody	Rituximab (Rituxan) [Genentech]	Not yet commenced
Monoclonal antibody	Daclizumab (Zenapax) [Biogen Idec/ PDL Biopharma Inc]	Not yet commenced

Source: www.clinicaltrials.gov (last accessed April 2009)

MONOCLONAL ANTIBODIES

Monoclonal antibodies are a group of substances which are designed specifically to attach to the surface of different cell types which are thought to be important in the disease process in MS. They are 'humanised', that is they are made to look similar to our own proteins to reduce the chance of our body trying to remove them. They still have the potential, however, to cause our immune system to generate neutralising antibodies to *them*!

Monoclonal antibodies are usually given via an intravenous drip unless otherwise stated. Allergic-type reactions can occur. Patients receiving monoclonal antibodies have a slightly increased risk of infection.

What do monoclonal antibodies have to do with treating MS?

An *antibody* is a protein produced naturally by cells from our immune system called B cells or B lymphocytes. An antibody can recognise and attach itself to a specific target (called an antigen) to which it has a complementary shape – like a key fitting into a lock. Monoclonal antibodies can be man-made to target and interfere with a very specific part of a disease process affecting the immune system in a beneficial way. In MS, neutralising antibody treatments are usually manufactured to target receptors on T or B cells (lymphocytes). In this way, they can reduce inflammation in the central nervous system and have a beneficial effect on MS.

Natalizumab (Tysabri) was the first licensed monoclonal antibody approved by NICE (the National Institute for Health and Clinical Excellence) for the treatment of rapidly evolving MS in the UK. There are several other monoclonal antibodies in the later stages of development (Phase 2 and Phase 3 studies) including alemtuzumab (Campath), rituximab (Rituxan) and daclizumab (Zenapax). More information about these and other drugs is given in Table 9.2.

Natalizumab (Tysabri)

I was told that a drug called Tysabri has big effects on MS but can have bad side effects. What does it do and is this true?

Natalizumab (Tysabri) is a manufactured monoclonal antibody licensed for use in the treatment of rapidly evolving MS. It prevents T-cells (lymphocytes) attaching to the inner lining of blood

Table 9.2 Monoclonal antibodies for MS in development

Antibody	Method of action	Phase 3 study dosing route and interval	Phase 2 study/duration	Side effects
Alemtuzumab	Targets on T and B cells and other white blood cells	5 daily doses intravenously (drip) with 3 days of steroids (drip) then 3 daily doses yearly (drip) or less	Significantly better than Rebif in range of clinical and MRI measures over three years	Thyroid disorders 11–30% Idiopathic thrombocytopaenic purpura 2.8%
Daclizumab	Target on activated T-cells	9 Subcutaneously (under the skin) fortnightly	When added to Interferon Beta significant reduction (72%) in new or enlarging plaques on MRI scans after 2 weeks treatment	Severe infections increase compared with placebo
Rituximab	Targets on some B cells	Intravenously (drip) at days 1 and 15	Reduced numbers of patients with relapses and reduced number of new plaques and enhancing plaques on MRI scans over 48 weeks	Urinary tract infections, sinusitis Angina/Heart attack (1 case) NB progressive multifocal leucoencephalopathy (PML) in other conditions

vessels, thereby stopping them from crossing the blood-brain barrier and passing into the central nervous system (brain and spinal cord).

Natalizumab appears to be more effective than the beta-interferons and glatiramer acetate in the treatment of MS. Clinical trials have demonstrated a greater than 60 per cent reduction in the number of relapses and a benefical effect on short-term disability in people treated with natalizumab compared to placebo ('dummy drug'). It is given once a month via an infusion ('a drip'). Natalizumab can occasionally cause a bad allergic reaction around the time of the infusion. Unfortunately, it can also cause a potentially fatal brain disorder called progressive multifocal leucoencephalopathy (PML). At the time of writing, the risk of PML is estimated to be 0.1 per cent (1 in 1,000). PML is caused by a virus called JC virus which most of us have in our bodies and which does not cause any problems as long as our immune system is working properly. However, in conditions that alter the immune system (such as HIV/AIDS) and with some monoclonal antibody treatments including natalizumab, the usually dormant JC virus can be reactivated and cause PML. This condition causes areas of inflammation within the brain which on MRI scanning may look different from those seen in MS. Confirmation of a diagnosis of PML usually requires a lumbar puncture.

Natalizumab is potentially teratogenic (harmful to the baby in the event of pregnancy) and it is therefore important to take contraceptive precautions and stop treatment if you are intending to get pregnant. If you are thinking of becoming pregnant it is important to discuss the management of your MS with your neurologist or MS nurse, so that any changes in treatment can be clearly planned and you can be closely monitored.

If your neurologist is considering treating you with natalizumab, he or she will discuss the latest information on the effectiveness of the medication and also potential side effects and risks including allergic reactions and PML. If you are started on natalizumab, your neurologist will monitor you carefully for any change in your condition which may raise the possibility of PML. This might include a change in your mood or personality or other neurological symptoms which are either not typical for MS or do not behave in a manner that would be expected in relapsing-remitting MS. If there is any concern about the possibility of PML, treatment will be stopped and an MRI scan and/or lumbar puncture performed. Treatment will only be restarted if test results are normal. If you have a bad allergic reaction to natalizumab at the time of an infusion, treatment will be stopped immediately and not restarted. Your neurologist will be able to discuss other treatment options if this occurs.

Alemtuzumab (Campath 1H, Mab-Campath)

I have heard a lot about Campath (alemtuzumab). What is it and how is it given?

Alemtuzumab (Campath-1H or Mab-Campath) is a monoclonal antibody that is currently licensed in the UK for the treatment of drug-resistant leukaemia. It targets and causes a long-term reduction in the number of T-cells (lymphocytes). Alemtuzumab appears to virtually 'switch off' ongoing inflammation in the brain and spinal cord. It is given via an infusion ('a drip') on five consecutive days that may then be repeated on three consecutive days at yearly intervals.

Can alemtuzumab help everyone with MS?

The short answer is 'no'. Alemtuzumab (Campath-1H or Mab-Campath) has been tested in people with both relapsing-remitting and secondary progressive MS with strikingly different results. In early studies, in carefully selected patients, almost all people with relapsing-remitting MS stabilised or improved with treatment, whereas most people with secondary progressive MS worsened despite treatment. These findings have led to a greater understanding about how disease-modifying drugs for MS should be used and to a theory that there may be a 'window of opportunity' during which powerful anti-inflammatory treatment may be very effective and, following which, treatment with these sorts of medications is futile. A clinical trial tested this hypothesis by studying people with very early MS (within three years of onset and with minimal disability). The study revealed that treatment with alemtuzumab led to more than a 70 per cent reduction in the number of relapses compared to beta-interferon 1a (Rebif 44). Furthermore, treatment with alemtuzumab led to a small improvement in the level of disability whereas those taking beta-interferon 1a worsened. One of the most important outcomes of this clinical trial may be the information it gives about whether aggressive early treatment of people with MS makes a long-term difference to their disability and prevents transition to the secondary phase of the condition. Long-term follow-up of the patients from this trial should give new insights into this vital issue.

Are there any risks with alemtuzumab?

As is the case with all aggressive treatments, the potential for improved beneficial effects must be weighed up against the risk of more serious potential side effects.

The side effects associated with alemtuzumab (Campath-1H or Mab-Campath) can be divided into those which occur at the time of the infusion and those which occur after completion of treatment. Common infusion-associated reactions include rash, headache, nausea, fatigue and chills. Alemtuzumab can also cause temporary re-emergence of previous symptoms. This distressing side effect is avoided by giving high dose steroids at the time of the infusion. Thyroid gland disorders occur in just over 20 per cent (around 1 in 4) of people receiving alemtuzumab – this problem can be picked up early with regular blood tests, but may require long-term treatment. Six people out of 223 (around 2.7 per cent) developed a condition called idio-pathic thrombocytopaenic purpura or ITP. This condition increases the risk of excessive bleeding and may be fatal if not detected early and treated. People receiving alemtuzumab are therefore given careful advice about the symptoms to watch out for – bruising and easy bleeding, for example when brushing their teeth and nosebleeds – in order that the condition may be diagnosed in good time and treated.

There also appears to be an increased risk of cancer. Alemtuzumab is potentially teratogenic (harmful to the baby in the event of pregnancy) so it is very important to take contraceptive precautions.

Alemtuzumab (Campath-1H or Mab-Campath) is not currently licensed for MS and its routine use is not recommended outside of clinical trials.

Rituximab

What does rituximab do, and what are the side effects?

Unlike most other monoclonal antibodies studied so far, rituximab targets a type of cell called a B lymphocyte or B-cell. B cells may have direct effects on the MS disease process through their production of antibodies but they can also stimulate the other type of lymphocyte (T-cells). Rituximab showed promise in a Phase 2 study of MS in which it appeared to be reducing the incidence of new brain plaques by over 90 per cent compared to placebo (dummy drug). Urinary tract infections and sinusitis were more common in the rituximab-treated group, although there was no difference in overall infection rates and most side effects occurred within 24 hours of the infusion (drip). Currently, there have been two cases of *progressive multi-focal leukoencephalopathy (PML)* who received rituximab as treatment for a condition called *systemic lupus erythematosis (SLE)*. It is not absolutely clear that rituximab was the cause of PML in these cases, as they had received other treatment, and PML is occasionally seen as a complication of SLE itself. Rituximab is also showing promise in treating neuromyelitis optica (NMO), another disorder which causes demyelination in the central nervous system.

Daclizumab

What about daclizumab?

Daclizumab was initially approved for use in prevention of kidney transplant rejection in the 1990s. Daclizumab attaches to the surface of T-cells (lymphocytes) and reduces their stimulation. In a Phase 2 study, which had not been fully published at the time this book went to press, daclizumab was given by subcutaneous injection under the skin every two weeks for 24 weeks in two doses. In the higher dose group, there was a reduction of almost three quarters in new brain plaques. Serious infections were more common in the daclizumab-treated group.

OTHER POTENTIAL DISEASE-MODIFYING DRUGS

Are there any other disease-modifying drugs in development?

Two injectable drugs being developed should be mentioned here: ATL1102 and BHT-3009.

ATL1102 (VLA-4 antisense oligonucleotide)
You will remember that natalizumab (Tysabri), an antibody, *blocks* T-cells (lymphocytes) from binding to the inner wall of blood vessels by attaching to a protein on the surface of the T-cells. ATL1102 achieves a similar effect by interfering with the message the body produces to *make* this protein. The effect is to reduce the numbers of targets for T-cells to attach to, thereby reducing the number of T-cells that get across the blood brain barrier.

A short-term Phase 2 study of ATL1102, when given as a subcutaneous (under the skin) injection twice weekly for 8 weeks, has shown significant reductions in new brain plaques on MRI scans. Side effects included injection site reactions and reduced platelet counts.

BHT-3009
BHT-3009 is a vaccine which causes production of a full-length replica of myelin basic protein (MBP), which is one of the major components of the myelin which coats and insulates nerve cells. By injecting this vaccine regularly, the intention is to make the immune system of people with MS 'tolerate' MBP better and therefore not react

against it. In the Phase 2 study, BHT-3009 was injected into the muscle two weeks apart for three doses then every four weeks until week 33. The preliminary report suggests that the positive effects on plaques on MRI scans are maintained for at least 8 months after the last injection is given and that patients did better than expected in terms of relapse rates over this period.

POTENTIAL ORAL (TABLET) TREATMENTS

All these drugs seem to be given through needles. Are any new drugs being developed as tablets for people like me who hate jabs?

There are indeed a number of drugs in development which are likely to be available in tablet form in the not too distant future. Some of them are already available on a limited basis or primarily for the treatment of other conditions. The list below may not be exhaustive, but it should give you some idea.

Cladribine
Cladribine reduces some types of T-cells and causes a temporary reduction in some types of B-cells too. The Phase 2 studies took place in the mid 1990s and at that stage it was administered via subcutaneous (under the skin) injections. The Phase 3 study required patients to take cladribine *tablets* in cycles of four to five days, two or four times in the first year and two cycles in the second year. Cladribine reduced relapse rates by 55–58 per cent compared with *placebo* (dummy drug).

Teriflunomide
Teriflunomide is given as a once daily tablet and is related to a drug called leflunomide which has been used in rheumatoid arthritis for around 10 years. It seems to interfere with the multiplication of activated T-cells (lymphocytes) but still allows a 'rescue' pathway to proceed so that T-cells can perform their normal functions.

Teriflunomide improved changes on MRI scans and the proportion of patients in whom MS progressed over a short period. Side effects of teriflunomide include sinusitis, loss of hair, nausea, pins and needles, diarrhoea, joint pain and abnormal liver blood tests and reduced numbers of neutrophils (white blood cells).

Fingolimod

Fingolimod is a man-made derivative of a naturally occurring fungus. It is given as a daily tablet. Fingolimod traps T-cells (lymphocytes) within lymph nodes thus stopping them getting into the brain and spinal cord. It also passes into the brain and acts on targets on the surface of nerve cells and oligodendrocytes, which produce the myelin insulation that coats nerve cells. In the Phase 2 study, in addition to improving changes on MRI scans, unusually it also significantly reduced relapse rates. Phase 3 trials are currently ongoing and patients are being monitored carefully for any heart, lung, eye or skin problems.

Initial results from a Phase 3 trial in which fingolimod was compared with beta-interferon (Avonex) showed that patients treated with fingolimod had between 38 per cent and 52 per cent fewer relapses than patients receiving Avonex. However, two patients who received high dose fingolimod died of complications relating to herpe virus infection and some patients treated with fingolimod developed skin cancer. There were also rare cases of macular oedema (swelling of the retina at the back of the eye).

Fumaric Acid (BG00012)

Fumarates reduce the numbers of T-cells (lymphocytes) by causing them to 'kill' themselves. Such drugs have been used in the treatment of psoriasis, a skin disorder, for over 20 years. The Phase 2 study in MS of a fumarate (BG00012) involved a tablet which was taken three times daily. Fumarate reduced the number of new plaques by two thirds when compared to placebo and improved other MRI outcomes. It was generally well tolerated. Flushing shortly after taking the drug, headache and abdominal pain were the most common side effects.

Laquinimod

Laquinimod seems to induce a beneficial change in the body's production of a type of immune cell that actually reduces inflammation. In the Phase 2 study with once daily tablets, the higher dose of laquinimod led to a 40 per cent reduction in the number of new plaques on MRI scans. Chest and joint pain occurred in the laquinimod group but not placebo group and raised liver blood tests were also more common with laquinimod. One case of a clot in the liver vein was noted in a patient with a pre-existing tendency to clot formation. This patient subsequently recovered.

I've heard that oestrogens may be beneficial in MS. Is this true?

Oestrogens are female sex hormones. It is known that the risk of relapses is reduced in women with MS during pregnancy – by about two-thirds in the last three months of pregnancy. Interestingly, this is better than treatment with beta-interferon (Avonex, Betaferon, Extavia, Rebif 22/44) and glatiramer acetate (Copaxone), but the benefit is only temporary. Unfortunately, the risk of relapses is increased in the three months following delivery to the extent that having children does not have any overall effect on relapse rate in MS. Nevertheless, this important finding has provided support for the notion that treatment with oestriol – an oestrogen produced only during pregnancy by the placenta – may be beneficial in MS. A Phase 2 clinical trial has produced encouraging initial results. At the time of writing, a Phase 3 clinical trial is ongoing and results are awaited.

Are statins helpful in MS?

Statins are currently used to treat raised cholesterol and to reduce the risk of heart attacks and strokes. They are given in tablet form and are generally well tolerated. There is experimental evidence to show that statins may be beneficial in MS but there are also some concerns they may be detrimental. A Phase 2 clinical trial has provided some encouraging initial results. Nevertheless, the potential role of statins in the treatment of MS is uncertain and Phase 3 clinical trials are needed in order to clarify matters.

Can cannabis alter the course of MS?

Cannabis-based drugs (cannabinoids) have been investigated in a number of clinical trials in an attempt to find out whether they may help some of the common *symptoms* encountered in MS including pain, spasticity and bladder problems. The largest of these clinical trials sought to determine whether tetrahydrocannabinol or THC (an active compound found in cannabis) helped spasticity but, unfortunately, results were inconclusive. However, the trial did provide some evidence that cannabinoids may have a beneficial disease-modifying effect in primary and secondary progressive MS, as patients who could walk when starting the trial could walk slightly more quickly at the end of the trial. Also, there were fewer relapses in patients receiving one form of cannabis-based medicine than in those taking placebo. A Phase 3 clinical trial investigating this possibility is ongoing and results are awaited.

You can read about research into cannabis-type drugs in Chapter 10.

I've heard that an anti-epilepsy drug may be helpful in MS – is this true?

There is experimental evidence to show that the anti-epilepsy drugs phenytoin (Epanutin) and lamotrigine (Lamictal) may reduce nerve cell (neuronal) loss in MS and may therefore be able to improve the course of the condition. A Phase 2 clinical trial of lamotrigine in secondary progressive MS has recently finished and the results should be available around the end of 2009.

10 | Research

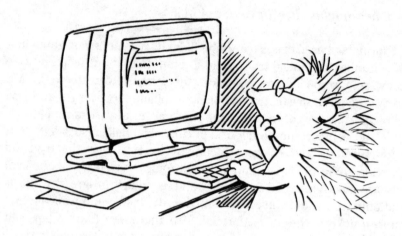

Research on the causes and ways of managing MS, including a large number of drug trials such as those discussed in the previous chapter, has increased dramatically in recent years. Much of the information that has advanced our understanding of MS has come from what is called 'basic research' – general knowledge of how the central nervous system works and, more recently, how susceptibility to the development of MS may be transmitted genetically.

MEDIA HYPE

Almost every week I read in the newspaper, or see on television, reports of scientists claiming to have discovered the 'cause' and the 'cure' of MS. No sooner has such a claim been made than there is another completely contradictory one. Why is this?

Multiple sclerosis is a very high profile condition and any new research findings may be considered newsworthy and published in newspapers or broadcast on radio and television. This information is sometimes presented in a way that is open to misinterpretation, giving the impression that a 'cure' for MS is imminent when this is simply not the case. This may lead to inappropriately raised hopes, disappointment and frustration for people with MS.

The following are useful tips when reading an article in a newspaper about new research in MS. Scrutinise it very carefully and try to judge whether the facts presented entirely justify the headline – journalists rarely understand the subject fully and are under pressure to produce exciting news items. Get a friend or colleague to cast a critical eye over the article and refer to other sources of information that may be less sensational in their reporting: the websites of the MS Society and MS Trust have up-to-date and reliable information provided by experts (see Appendix 1). Try to maintain a healthy scepticism for any report of a 'breakthrough', particularly if this is the opinion of a person or an organisation that may have a vested interest in promoting the research. Articles which use emotive language such as 'hope' should also be viewed with caution.

When considering specific reports of new treatments in MS, it is important to understand what does, and what does not, constitute robust evidence of benefit. Keep a mental checklist of the sorts of things to look out for. In particular, be very wary of any anecdotal reports concerning a small number of people's individual experiences of a novel therapy.

Anyone may improve while taking treatment if they believe it to be effective – this is known as a 'non-specific placebo effect'. Phase 3 clinical trials are designed to try and eliminate these sorts of problems and are needed before a new drug can get a licence for use and become available for prescription. Phase 3 clinical trials typically involve very large numbers of people and have the following features:

- They are placebo-controlled – this means the drug is compared to a placebo ('dummy drug'). This is necessary to help ensure the drug can be shown to have a specific benefit above the non-specific effects of a placebo.

- They are randomised – this means a person cannot choose whether they get the new drug or a placebo.

- They are *double-blinded* – this means neither the person nor the doctor knows whether the person is receiving the new drug or a placebo.

When considering the results of a clinical trial, it is also important to check whether it has actually been completed. This may seem obvious but sometimes an ongoing clinical trial is reported in order to raise its profile and recruit suitable participants – the report may include reasons why it has been organised and give the impression the treatment is effective when it is not actually known for sure whether it is. Indeed, finding out whether or not a treatment will be effective is usually the reason the clinical trial is being conducted in the first place.

Finally, it is always important to remain positive. There is a great deal of high quality research and there are many clinical trials in progress. It seems inevitable this will lead to a better understanding of MS and improved treatments in the future.

TYPES OF RESEARCH

What are the specific areas of research in MS at the moment?

There are five kinds of research being undertaken in MS at present:

- **Epidemiological research** is the study of the geographical distribution and patterns of MS – it involves asking questions about whether MS is more common in one area than another, or is decreasing or increasing in a particular population over time, and what factors might explain these differences.

- **'Case-control' studies.** These are studies that investigate the backgrounds of people. Individual people with MS are compared with those without the condition who are of similar age and gender and who have other things in common – in an attempt to identify factors that may be implicated in the cause of MS. One of the problems of this kind of research is that it has to be done retrospectively, relying on people's memories, and may therefore be an unreliable source of information.

- **Laboratory-based research** usually involves working with samples of blood or other tissues from people with MS. It tends to focus on questions related to the development of MS, such as how and why it affects the central nervous system and what are the possible genetic differences between people with and without MS. Sometimes inducing illnesses similar to MS in animals can give us important information regarding treatments that may alter the course of the illness, by protecting nerve cells from injury and death.

- **Clinical research** focuses on the 'natural development' of MS by investigating particular symptoms and signs that develop in people over time, and the consequences these may have on their ability to function in everyday life. It can also address questions about the effectiveness and safety of potential new therapies for MS, undertaken through clinical trials.

- **Applied research** may involve, for example, the investigation of how physiotherapy or speech therapy or other interventions can reduce the impact of symptoms, or how psychological support or counselling may help people to manage their symptoms better.

GENETICS

Scientists say that they have recently discovered 'the MS gene'. What does that mean for me and for my condition?

We have already discussed that genetic factors account for only about one third of a person's risk of developing MS. There are regular stories in the media with headlines suggesting that a new gene for MS has been discovered. These stories are usually a little exaggerated. A number of genes have been consistently shown to be found more frequently in people with MS than people without the condition. The strongest association is with a collection of genes that contain the information necessary to produce the proteins on the surface of white blood cells, including T and B cells (lymphocytes). These are called human leucocyte antigens (HLA), and can be considered similar to the proteins found on red blood cells that underlie ABO blood groups. One particular HLA group, HLA DR (2) 15, has been consistently shown to be associated with an increased risk of getting MS. This HLA type is actually very common – more than 50 per cent (1 in 2) of people in the UK have it and they are about five times more likely to have or develop MS than people who do not.

It isn't generally felt to be useful to test for this HLA variant, however, as the results wouldn't really be that helpful. This is because a person would still be much more likely never to develop MS even if they were found to be HLA DR (2) 15 'positive'. Since there is no treatment at present that can be offered to prevent MS in people at higher risk of developing it, the identification of these 'at risk' people is of no great usefulness.

All of the evidence suggests that there must be at least five genes involved in determining a person's individual risk of getting MS. To complicate things further, the genes responsible are likely to differ from person to person. Even if we had the ability to screen a person's individual DNA, and we knew all of the genes that play a role in MS and how they applied to that person, we would still only be able to give them an age-adjusted estimated risk of having or developing MS, because environmental factors and luck also play a major role.

Does all this research into the genetics of MS mean that scientists will find a cure for MS, like they have for cystic fibrosis?

Cystic fibrosis is caused by a single defective gene. Fortunately, it has been possible to work out how this gene works and, as a consequence, to develop a treatment for the condition. MS is a completely different disease with a much more complex genetic basis. It probably involves five or more genes, each of which has only a small effect on the risk of getting MS. Furthermore, it seems very likely there are other genes that determine the severity of the condition once it develops. It is therefore going to be much more difficult to find a cure for MS than is has been for cystic fibrosis.

CLINICAL TRIALS

I keep hearing about clinical trials of new drugs in MS. What is a clinical trial?

A clinical trial may be considered to be a controlled experiment which tests a hypothesis (for example, is the drug beneficial in MS?). Clinical trials are designed to find out whether there is a difference between the effect of treatment with a new drug and the effect of treatment with a placebo ('dummy drug') or other standard medication. This treatment effect is known as the primary outcome measure. In clinical trials of potential disease-modifying drugs in MS, the primary outcome is usually some measure of relapses or disability. It is generally accepted that if the difference in the primary outcome measure between the new drug and placebo may have arisen as a chance result less than 1 in 20 times, then it is statistically significant. This is denoted as a probability (P) value of less than 0.05 (1 in 20).

This is usually written as $P<0.05$. However, it is always important to remember that even if a difference is of statistical significance, it does not necessarily mean it is of *clinical* significance – the difference may be quite small and of no meaningful benefit.

The clinical trials required to get a new drug licensed for use typically involve hundreds of people and are usually randomised, blinded and placebo-controlled. Randomisation means that people are randomly allocated to either the new drug or placebo. This helps to balance out the treatment groups so that they are similar in terms of age, gender, type and duration of MS. It also means that the doctor and person with MS will not have any control over which treatment is allocated. Blinding (or masking) means neither the doctor nor the person with MS knows whether they are receiving the new drug or placebo. Placebo-controlled means that the new drug needs to show an actual benefit over and above that shown by a placebo: it is well recognised that people with MS can improve on placebo even though it does not contain any active ingredients. This is known as 'the placebo effect'.

Are there many ongoing clinical trials in MS?

The MS Society calculated that by mid 2008 there were 92 ongoing clinical trials, examining 62 different agents. Of these 92 trials, 80 included people with relapsing-remitting MS, 33 with secondary progressive MS and 17 with primary progressive MS. There were seven trials which recruited people with clinically isolated syndromes. For the latest information about clinical trials, please see the websites of the MS Society, MS Trust or go to www.clinicaltrials.gov.

What is the difference between a Phase 1 and a Phase 2 clinical trial? And are there any other 'Phases'?

Phase 1 clinical trials are usually conducted on small numbers of healthy volunteers. They are designed to check there are no common and unexpected side effects as this is the first time a new drug may have been used on humans. Phase 2 clinical trials are usually conducted on small numbers of people with the condition under investigation. They are designed to find out whether there is any prospect that the new drug is effective, and to check again that there are no common side effects. If the results of Phase 1 and 2 clinical trials are encouraging, Phase 3 clinical trials are then conducted. These typically include very large numbers of people and are usually randomised, double-blinded and placebo-controlled (see above). Phase 3 clinical trials are needed to confirm that the new drug under investigation is both effective and safe. They also provide evidence that will enable the regulatory authorities to decide whether the new drug should be licensed for use and available for prescription. Phase 4 studies are extensions of Phase 3 clinical trials and involve the continued monitoring of people on the new drug to ensure there are no other unexpected or rare side effects that may only become apparent after the drug is in widespread use.

The total period from Phase 1 studies to the licensing of a drug may take over 20 years. Unfortunately, many drugs that show early promise – and are reported about enthusiastically at the time – may fall by the wayside at a later stage, never to be heard of again. Nevertheless, there are so many ongoing clinical trials in MS it seems inevitable that more effective drug treatments will become available in future years.

I am keen to participate in clinical trials in order to get the chance of taking a new drug. How do I make sure I receive the new drug?

Whether or not you receive a new drug depends upon the clinical trial design. A 'parallel group' study keeps people in the same group throughout the whole of the study. Typically, people are allocated the new drug or placebo ('dummy drug') in equal numbers and on a random basis – this means you will have a 50 per cent (1 in 2) chance of receiving the new drug. You will not have any choice or know whether you are receiving the new drug, or placebo, until after the end of the clinical trial. Some studies allow more people to be allocated the new drug than placebo – this means you will have greater than 1 in 2 chance of receiving the new drug but there is still no guarantee. A crossover study, as the name suggests, allows people to switch from the initial treatment they were allocated to the other treatment during the trial period. People in a crossover study will therefore receive the new drug at some stage during the trial but they will not know when. Some clinical trials have an open-label extension phase. This means people will be offered the new drug at trial completion in order that more information can be obtained about its long-term safety. Open-label means that both you and your doctor will know you are receiving the new drug.

It is very important to discuss all these issues with your doctor before you agree to take part in a clinical trial. It is also important to establish whether or not the new drug may be available to you when the trial is completed in order to avoid disappointment.

Will I have to pay for the drugs I receive in a clinical trial?

No – medications are provided free of charge during the period of the study. You should not be out of pocket for participating in a clinical trial. If a study has a commercial sponsor, such as a pharmaceutical company, your travel expenses and other necessary costs will usually be reimbursed. You should ask about this before agreeing to participate in a study.

How do I get to participate in clinical trials of new drugs?

The best way is to ask your neurologist or MS nurse what clinical trials are taking place in your area. If you are eligible to be recruited to an ongoing clinical trial you may be invited to participate. If not, your name can be put on a list of potentially suitable candidates for future clinical trials. If you discover a clinical trial that is being conducted elsewhere, it is sensible to ask your neurologist about this in order to find out whether you are eligible and if there may be any concerns about you taking part. This is particularly important in trials of disease-modifying drugs.

POTENTIAL TREATMENTS FOR SYMPTOMS

Although it is tempting to believe claims in the media and on the internet regarding new treatments in MS, it is always important to ask, *'Show me the evidence'*. Treatments should have demonstrated a benefit in carefully conducted clinical trials and to minimise the chance of either a positive result by a fluke or an exaggeration of the benefit, the trial should have a large enough number of patients. Patients should receive their treatment randomly and not because of other factors such as gender, age, or date of birth, the trial should contain a dummy placebo tablet or pretend 'sham' intervention where the patient thinks they could have had the 'real thing' and the doctors and patients should not know which intervention the patients actually received. This is the basis of the randomised double-blind placebo-controlled trial.

We have indicated what trials, if any, have been undertaken for a number of treatments listed below for which there are advocates and these are easy to find on the internet. Remember in these circumstances always ask, *'Show me the evidence!'*

> *I have heard a lot about low dose naltrexone (LDN). What is it and does it work for MS?*

Naltrexone in high doses (50 mg to 100 mg per day) blocks the targets (receptors) for opioids such as codeine, morphine and heroin. It has been used in people with addiction to these drugs or to alcohol. In lower doses however (less than or equal to 5 mg per day) naltrexone has a stimulating effect on opioid receptors, leading to a sustained release of the body's own opioids such as beta-endorphins, which have effects on pain, mood, hormones, appetite and when released by lymphocytes, are anti-inflammatory. These widespread effects have led to the use of LDN to treat a number of symptoms such as bladder dysfunction, fatigue and spasticity, in a number of different conditions.

Although there have been many claims for the benefits of naltrexone, the controlled trials evidence to date in MS is sparse. The largest fully published trial to date of 40 patients with primary progressive MS was open-label, that is all patients knew they were receiving LDN. This type of trial tends to over estimate the effect of a treatment. Nevertheless, there was an increase in pain, no change in disability, fatigue, quality of life and a possible reduction in spasticity. A further study, not fully published when this book went to press, of 80 patients over 8 weeks of treatment which was double-blinded and placebo-controlled, suggested improvements in some non-physical quality of life outcomes, but requires scrutiny in a peer-reviewed journal.

Some recent work has suggested that LDN may prevent or delay the onset of the animal model of MS, and reduce its severity. In summary, all of these results require replication in larger studies before any conclusions about any efficacy of LDN can be reached.

I have heard about the 'Cari Loder regime'. What is this and does it work?

Cari Loder is a person with MS who developed a treatment regime consisting of lofepramine (an antidepressant), phenylalanine (an essential amino acid, one of the building blocks for proteins which can only be obtained through the diet and is contained in, for example, cola) and vitamin B12. She wrote a book about her experiences after taking this treatment combination.

A formal clinical trial was conducted to establish whether or not this treatment regime had significant benefits in people with MS. All patients received a vitamin B12 injection weekly, and either lofepramine and L-phenylalanine twice daily, or matching placebo tablets.

Both groups had a small reduction in disability. Patients who received all three treatments had a further very small improvement over those who only received vitamin B12. The authors concluded that further studies were needed to examine how the benefit arose, but that the additional benefit over vitamin B12 was probably clinically insignificant and that the results did not support the widespread use of this combination.

I have heard about a new treatment called Fampridine.
What can you tell me about it?

Fampridine (4-aminopyridine) is a drug that can improve the passage of nerve impulses down damaged neurons (nerve cells). A Phase 3 clinical trial has shown it may improve mobility and quality of life. It also appears to be relatively well tolerated. It is important to appreciate this drug is a symptomatic treatment – it is not a disease-modifying drug and will not alter the course of the condition. It is likely the company involved in the drug's development will apply for regulatory approval, but the outcome of this is difficult to predict.

CANNABIS-BASED MEDICINES

Cannabinoids, derived from the cannabis plant or manufactured synthetically, can be delivered in a number of different ways for recreational as well as medicinal use. In order to differentiate between illegal 'street' cannabis, which varies in strength, purity and proportions of different cannabinoids, and pharmaceutical standard products, manufactured with the same rigour as any other 'prescription drug', we will refer to the former as 'cannabis' and the latter as 'cannabis-based medicines', whether they are made from cannabis plant or synthetically manufactured.

Does cannabis work for MS?

This question is not as easy to answer as it may sound and there are a number of factors to take into account when trying to answer it! Some of these factors are explored more fully in the answers below. The short answer is that when cannabis-based medicines have been formally studied in clinical trials, they may have shown some promise but, so far, the results have been conflicting and inconsistent. At present, therefore, the drug licensing body in the UK, the Medicines Health and Regulatory Authority (MHRA) has yet to receive sufficient and consistent enough evidence of the benefit of a cannabis-based medicine to license one for the treatment of symptoms of MS. However, one cannabis-based medicine (Sativex) has received a preliminary licence for use in Canada.

Anecdotal evidence from people who smoke cannabis illegally, and claim that it may be beneficial, is not sufficient to recommend its use. In addition to its illegality, its variation in strength, purity and proportions of different cannabinoids between batches makes it difficult to measure doses. People will often say that they either under-estimate the dose (in which case any perceived beneficial effects are less than expected) or over-estimate it (in which case they may develop a number of unpleasant side effects). When smoked, cannabis is usually cut with tobacco, so the usual concerns about health risks including development of cancer apply.

I keep reading about different types of cannabis-based medicine being studied for MS? Sometimes the articles talk about a spray, other times, tablets. What is the difference and why not just test one?

Cannabinoids are chemical compounds which share a similar structure. They can be sourced in three ways, as follows:

1. Cannabis plants contain over 60 cannabinoids, often in different proportions. The two most common are delta-9-tetrahydrocannabinol (THC), which is the most studied cannabinoid and the one associated with a number of the well-known psychological effects, and cannabidiol (CBD) which can reduce some of the side effects of THC by delaying its breakdown in the liver. CBD also has some potential

therapeutic properties of its own, such as pain relief. Sativex, a cannabis-based medicine in liquid form derived from plants, is sprayed on the inside of the cheek. It contains THC and CBD in roughly equal proportions.

❷ Cannabinoids can be man-made and a synthetic version of THC (Nabilone) is actually licensed for use in the UK, but for post-operative nausea and vomiting in people receiving chemotherapy, *not* for MS. Some doctors will consider prescribing Nabilone off-licence for people who have found symptomatic benefit from cannabis, though, anecdotally, it does not seem to be as effective as cannabis plant.

❸ The human body has a natural 'endocannabinoid' system which is involved in a number of system, both within and outside of the nervous system. Although there are no licensed drugs which manipulate the endocannabinoid system, it is obviously an attractive focus for further research.

If cannabis is eaten or cannabis-based medicines are taken as tablets, their absorption into the bloodstream depends upon the amount of food within the stomach. If it is delayed, then the liver inactivates a variable proportion of the drug before it gets into the nervous system and exerts an effect. This makes the dosing of cannabis-based medicines difficult. The manufacturers of Sativex have tried to overcome this variability by delivering it directly into the main blood circulation via the veins in the mouth. Of course, delivery of a drug in this way on a long-term basis can cause irritation and local side effects.

It is still not clear whether a single cannabinoid or a mixture is best for treating symptoms of MS, or whether synthetic cannabinoids are best, or the mixture of 'minor' cannabinoids in cannabis-based medicines made from cannabis plants have a benefit. For these reasons there a number of different cannabis-based medicines in development, some synthetic, some plant derived, some with single cannabinoids, and others with combinations in varying proportions.

The possibility that cannabis-based drugs may have a disease-modifying effect is currently under investigation and clinical trial results are awaited. The effects of cannibinoids on progression of disability in MS are currently being assessed in the CUPID study which is following up 500 patients with progressive MS over 3 years.

What is the main substance in cannabis that doctors are concerned with, and what effects does it have?

Cannabinoids are a group of substances found in cannabis. The major cannabinoids are tetrahydrocannabinol (THC) and cannabidiol (CBD). THC is thought to be the main psychoactive component that causes the 'high' (euphoria) experienced by cannabis users. THC, either in its natural or synthetic forms, is the cannabinoid used in clinical trials. It can be given on its own or in combination with CBD to minimise unwanted side effects.

Can the way cannabis is taken affect the way it works?

Yes. When cannabis is taken for recreational use it is usually smoked. The active substances contained in cannabis (cannabinoids) are absorbed through the lungs into the bloodstream then to the brain. Because it is absorbed very rapidly via this route, cannabis users are often able to vary its effects by altering how much they inhale. Unfortunately, inhaling burnt cannabis cut with tobacco can cause lung cancer, so this is not an appropriate mode of administration for medicinal use.

Although cannabis can be eaten or taken in tablet form, it is absorbed more slowly through the stomach than the lungs and it is therefore more difficult to judge the right amount to take. It is for these reasons that other ways of taking cannabis-based medicines have been developed, or are under development, including oral sprays and inhalers.

When taken by mouth, cannabis is absorbed from the gut, but the speed at which it is absorbed depends upon how full your stomach is at the time it is taken. After absorption, it enters the bloodstream and passes into the liver where it is partly broken down. It then enters the main bloodstream and is taken to the nervous system and the rest of the body.

Both of these factors mean that when cannabis is taken by mouth, the actual amount which reaches the brain, and the speed with which it reaches it, can vary between doses.

STEM CELL THERAPY

I've heard about stem cell therapy. What can you tell me about this?

Stem cell therapy has huge potential in the treatment of MS. This is because stem cells are capable of renewing themselves and changing into other cells including those that make myelin (oligodendrocytes). This opens up the exciting prospect of stem cell therapy promoting remyelination (renewing myelin) or repairing the malfunctioning immune system that causes inflammation in the brain and spinal cord.

Stem cell therapy is a rather complex subject as there are a number of different stem cell types and forms of therapy to consider. Embryonic stem cells are obtained from a human embryo or fetus and are capable of changing into any cell type – these sorts of stem cells have the most potential but there are important ethical issues concerning how they are obtained. Adult stem cells can only change into a limited number of different cell types – although they are not as capable as embryonic stem cells, they are relatively easy to obtain from bone marrow and umbilical cord blood.

One important consideration in stem cell therapy is how to get stem cells to the parts of the brain and spinal cord damaged in MS. This is a very tricky proposition because MS causes multiple areas of damage throughout the central nervous system. Although direct transplantation of stem cells into the brain or spinal cord might be an option in a person with one particularly severe area of damage, this is unlikely to be feasible in the vast majority of people with MS. It is therefore very encouraging that early research indicates stem cells may be able to find their own way to damaged parts of the central nervous system if injected into the bloodstream. Other forms of stem cell therapy seek to replace a malfunctioning immune system in the hope this will prevent further damage to the central nervous system and perhaps allow repair to take place. Autologous bone marrow transplantation is one example of this form of stem cell therapy – it involves destroying a person's immune system using powerful chemotherapy and then replacing it using the person's own preserved bone marrow stem cells. This is a very controversial treatment because it has a significant mortality (death) rate.

Unfortunately, there are a number of other problems that must be overcome before stem cell therapy can be shown to be both effective and safe. These include how to ensure stem cells survive once they have been transplanted, how to stop them renewing themselves too much and causing cancer, and how to avoid infection. Despite all these concerns, stem cell therapy shows great promise and seems to be one of the best hopes of finding a way to stop – or even reverse – the damage caused by MS.

I'm thinking about paying to have stem cell therapy abroad. What do you think?

Although stem cell therapy has great potential, research is still at a very early stage. So the potential risks of treatment, including cancer and infections, are cause for concern. Clinical trials are always needed to confirm the benefits and safety of any new treatment, and stem cell therapy is no exception. At present, there are no clinical trial results to support the routine use of stem cell therapy in MS.

Despite all these unresolved issues, a number of commercial companies are offering stem cell therapy directly to people with MS. It is concerning that many people who have received treatment have not been properly assessed neurologically, or with MRI scanning, either before or after treatment. Rigorous monitoring is needed in order to show benefits and to detect harmful side effects. The therapies on offer are usually very expensive. The Association of British Neurologists – an organisation that represents neurologists in the UK – has stated stem cell therapy should not take place outside of the confines of a clinical trial. It strongly advises people considering stem cell therapy to discuss this with their neurologist before proceeding in order to ensure they know about the reputation of the establishment offering treatment.

11 | Complementary therapies and MS

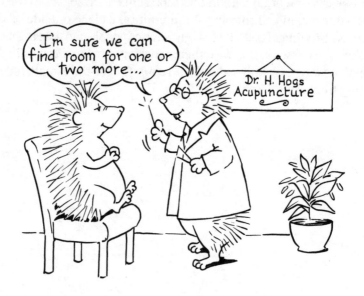

When there is no current scientifically-accepted cure for a disease, it is understandable that many people want to explore novel or less conventional approaches. Whereas, at one time, the medical establishment was very suspicious of so-called 'alternative' therapies, it is an increasingly widely held view that if you find something that may help your symptoms without doing any harm, it is reasonable to try it. Some doctors would argue however that before they can be recommended, complementary therapies should be subjected to the same rigorous trials and assessments as any conventional drug or therapy. *Complementary therapies* should be exactly that, treatments explored at the same time as a person is being cared for by their medical team, rather than used as an alternative to the treatment they receive from healthcare professionals.

Complementary therapies are very varied in nature, and are often based on different, and sometimes conflicting, views of how the body – and mind – operates. One distinguishing characteristic of these treatments is their focus on the whole person and the use of the body's own healing powers to meet the challenges of disease. Partly because of the broad focus of such therapies and their gearing to individuals as much as to diseases, they are very difficult to evaluate in formal scientific terms. Indeed, many complementary therapies have not yet been scientifically studied even though their practitioners and patients may have a very high opinion of their value.

WHERE TO GO

How can I find a practitioner in a particular complementary therapy?

There are many different ways in which you can track down a reputable practitioner of a particular complementary therapy. The vast majority of practitioners within the area of complementary therapy are excellent but (as in any profession) some individuals will not practise to the same high standards. It is therefore very important to find someone you can trust. The best and most reliable way is by word of mouth: if someone you know has first-hand experience of a practitioner in a therapy area which interests you, and can make a positive recommendation, this is probably worth pursuing.

The Internet is also a good source of information about complementary therapies and therapists, but not all the information is reliable. Once you have identified a treatment in which you are interested, find out if therapists in this area have a professional body with which they may be registered. If this is the case, track down the practitioners in your area via their professional body, in order to ensure the person you contact is appropriately qualified and registered. The addresses of some of these professional bodies are given in Appendix 1.

Once you have identified the practitioners in your area, give them a ring and ask questions about their therapies, the evidence for their use, potential side effects and the overall service they provide. Don't be afraid to ask for references and follow these up before making an appointment. You may also find it is worth asking others – perhaps people in your local MS Society branch or your MS nurse or GP – they may know of a reputable local therapist or centre where you can access complementary therapies more easily.

There seem to be a lot of benefits from complementary therapies. Even my doctor has mentioned some of the methods available. But who will pay for it?

Complementary therapies are not routinely available on the NHS. It is sometimes possible to have limited sessions of therapies such as acupuncture or reflexology through your local healthcare team if there are qualified practitioners of these therapies within the team and you meet the criteria for referral. It is always worth discussing this option with your GP, physiotherapist or MS nurse. However, it is most likely you will have to fund the treatment yourself. If this is a problem, it may be worth approaching your local branch of the MS Society as they can sometimes provide help with funding or may have access to certain treatments at reduced cost. Your MS nurse may also be able to point you in the direction of a local charity which might allow you to receive treatment at a lower cost than if you organised your treatment directly with the practitioner.

DIFFERENT COMPLEMENTARY THERAPIES

There has been a lot of publicity recently about people with MS using cannabis to help reduce spasticity and pain. If it can help me, I would like to try it. How can I obtain it?

A necdotal evidence suggests that some people with MS have found cannabis can help a variety of symptoms including spasticity and pain. But clinical trials of cannabis-based medicines have so far not been able to provide objective evidence that it has a consistent and significant benefit.

Cannabis is illegal and has recently been reclassified as a Class B drug, which means the maximum penalty for possession is five years in prison and an unlimited fine. We cannot therefore recommend anyone to use cannabis illegally. Cannabis obtained 'on the street' is also more likely to be mixed with contaminants and to be of unknown quality and concentration, and so may cause harm even in small doses.

Some people with MS have been able to obtain a prescription for a cannabis-based medicine from their GP if recommended by their neurologist – this tends to be for people with chronic nerve pain which has not improved with a number of standard medications. The process by which your GP may obtain a cannabis-based medicine can be quite lengthy and is not always successful.

One particular cannabis derivative is nabilone (Marinol). This is a synthetic cannabinoid licensed for use in the treatment of nausea and vomiting in people receiving chemotherapy. Unfortunately, there are usually prescribing restrictions imposed on its use and, again, informal feedback indicates this is not particularly effective or well tolerated in people with MS. Sativex is a cannabinoid (THC/CBD combination) given by oral spray. It is currently unlicensed and there are usually prescribing restrictions that limit its availability. This is likely to remain the case pending the results of ongoing clinical trials. More information about cannabinoid drugs in development can be found in Chapter 10.

There have been many TV documentaries and newspaper stories written about revolutionary new therapies for MS. What do you think of them?

MS is a disease which is life-long, currently has no cure and which varies enormously both between individuals and over time, for each individual. The majority of people experience periods of relatively good health followed by episodes where symptoms become more troublesome. This inevitably and understandably means that most people with MS and their families experience a great deal of anxiety and uncertainty in their lives.

The 'ups and downs' in symptoms over time make people with MS and their families, particularly vulnerable to false claims of 'miracle cures' and revolutionary new treatments. This difficulty arises because someone with MS can spontaneously improve, and if this happens to coincide with taking a new treatment it can be all too easy to assume that the improvement is due to the treatment. This is why it is so important for any new drug to be properly tested in a clinical trial to prove that it works better than a *placebo* ('dummy drug') or other standard treatment. Be sceptical about reports which use emotive language like 'hope' however tempting it is to believe the headline at face value.

If a new treatment does stand up to scientific testing and is shown to be effective for people with MS, it is likely to be licensed for use by the regulatory authorities and available for prescription. However, restrictions on its prescription may apply. If you see an article or documentary about a new drug for MS that you think may be helpful for you then contact your MS nurse or neurologist and discuss it with them. Alternatively, have a look on the MS Society or MS Trust websites as they will always provide balanced advice about any new treatments which are in the news.

What are all these new therapies?

Research into MS is a very active field and can be categorised into three main areas:

- Research into modifying the course of the disease;
- Research into symptom management;
- Research into understanding the nature of MS better so that we can target future treatments more appropriately.

Any of these areas of research can provide potential new therapies or novel management strategies.

The nature of research means that it is not possible to list all the new therapies which are being investigated at any one time. Unfortunately, many potential therapies will not make the grade and prove not to be effective or safe enough to be used in MS. A few will go on and prove to be clinically effective, well tolerated and safe. After years of clinical trials, these new drugs may make it through to the front line of care where they may be available for use, although prescribing restrictions may apply.

A great deal of information about potential new therapies is available on the internet, but not all of it is reliable. The MS Society and MS Trust are both very good sources of information (see Appendix 1 for details). Another useful source of information is the Association of the British Pharmaceutical Industry (ABPI) which publishes a booklet about MS that can be downloaded from the website. It also contains information about new therapies in development.

Some of my friends with MS have told me to try complementary therapies. Can you list some that are available?

It is estimated that between 50 per cent (1 in 2) and 75 per cent (3 out of 4) of people with MS use complementary therapies to help them manage their condition more effectively. In 2003, NICE (the

National Institute for Health and Clinical Excellence) published guidelines setting out the care people with MS should receive – these guidelines were the first to include reference to the use of complementary therapies. While cautioning that there is insufficient evidence to make any firm recommendations, NICE lists reflexology, massage, t'ai chi, fish oils, magnetic field therapy, neural therapy and multi-modal therapy as being potentially useful. If you want to find out more about whether any of these treatments could help, don't hesitate to talk to your MS nurse, neurologist or GP who should be able to give you more information.

Should I try acupuncture?

In its traditional form, acupuncture is based on the idea that energy (chi or qi) flows round the body through channels called meridians which become blocked at times of illness and stress. Acupuncturists insert very fine needles at key points on these meridians to unblock energy flows and help restore health. Acupressure (often known as *shiatzu*) works on a similar principle, but uses pressure from fingers or thumbs at these energy points. The results of some scientific studies suggest that in certain circumstances acupuncture does appear to relieve pain (although acupuncturists claim more general benefits). Trials of acupuncture are often criticised as it is notoriously difficult to make them truly placebo-controlled and positive effects may only be short-term. It would be wise to seek a diagnosis of any pain from your GP or neurologist, before undertaking such a treatment, in case there are other causes that need to be treated.

I used to do yoga when I was much younger. Would it be a good thing to take it up again now I have been diagnosed with MS?

Yoga is widely used by many people with MS, and there are now teachers and specialist centres where it is available. From a practical point of view, yoga can be seen as providing a form of exercise, which is known to be helpful in keeping your muscles working, as well as a way of calming of the mind in order to help counter depression, stress and fatigue. One advantage of yoga is that, in addition to its emphasis on slow movement, peace and calm, you can undertake the exercises at home once you have received training. Its emphasis on deep and controlled breathing can also be helpful, particularly if your posture is not what it should be, or if you are sitting for long periods.

The main concern with yoga for MS is that you should work well within your limitations in a relaxed way, and be careful not to push yourself too far as this may increase fatigue. If you have had physiotherapy, it may be an idea to consult your physiotherapist about starting yoga. You can obtain more information about yoga from the Yoga for Healthcare Education Trust or people with MS and other conditions, or from the Royal London Homeopathic Hospital (Yoga Biomedical Trust) (see Appendix 1).

I think I would really enjoy having aromatherapy. But is it safe for me?

Yes. Aromatherapy is a massage with specific oils. The oils used are called 'essential oils'. They are very concentrated and should always be used with a carrier oil (such as almond oil) during massage. They must not be taken by mouth. Some of the oils should not be used if you are pregnant or have epilepsy; it is crucial that you let your aromatherapist know if there is any cause for concern. Massage is potentially valuable, not only for relaxing muscles and reducing spasticity, but also for promoting a general sense of well-being. It is very important that you check what form of massage the therapist is offering, and ensure that the therapist has been well trained and, above all, knows about MS. This is because some forms of massage are very vigorous and seek to realign the musculature of the body. These realigning forms of massage should be avoided in people with MS. However, most aromatherapists use much gentler forms of massage.

What is reflexology?

Reflexology is a type of therapy based on the idea that energy and other flows in the body are linked to key points in the feet, providing a 'map' of key organs and systems in the body. It is believed that problems in all parts of the body can be identified and indeed treated through manipulating the feet. Some people with MS have indicated that they have found reflexology helpful and relaxing even though there is no formal evidence that it affects the course of MS, or any major symptoms of the condition. However, as a relaxing form of therapy, it may benefit some people with MS.

What is the difference between osteopathy and chiropractic?
They sound like the same thing to me.

Osteopathy is a relatively long-standing, well regulated and trained profession compared to some other complementary therapy disciplines. All practitioners must be registered with the General Osteopathic Council (see Appendix 1). Osteopaths manipulate bones, muscles and tissues to enhance well-being, particularly by working with the skeletal structures and joints. Treatment may also involve established medical diagnostic procedures (including X-rays and blood tests), joint manipulation, rhythmic exercise and stretching. Osteopathy can improve mobility in the spine and affected joints.

Chiropractic is a long-standing approach founded on a particular view of the way in which the human body works and may be managed. As in osteopathy, practitioners manipulate the bones, muscles and tissues, especially around the spine. Practitioners can use a variety of techniques and a course of treatment is usually composed of short sessions spaced out over several months. Chiropractic recommends itself particularly for back pain and persistent headaches. In very rare instances, manipulation of the spinal column can cause lasting damage, so always ensure you consult a qualified chiropractor and that you discuss your MS fully before any treatment begins.

What is your opinion about homeopathy as a treatment for MS?

Homeopathy is based on the notion that 'like cures like' – it involves the use of very dilute substances (usually in the form of tablets or drops). A homeopathic practitioner takes a holistic view of anyone they see, taking into account personality, temperament and lifestyle as well as the medical diagnosis and symptoms experienced, before recommending a particular treatment.

There is no scientific research that shows whether or not homeopathy can help people with MS. Although there is anecdotal evidence that some people find homeopathic treatment beneficial, it is not known whether this is simply a placebo effect – it is well recognised that people with MS may benefit from an inactive dummy drug (placebo) if they believe it to be effective. It seems reasonable for a person who feels strongly they want to try homeopathy, to go ahead, so long as they can find a reputable practitioner and are happy it is not going to cause them any harm and that it is not going to cost more than they are willing (or able) to pay.

What about oxygen therapy?

Oxygen therapy, or hyperbaric oxygen (HBO), is a form of treatment offered by MS resource centres around the country. It involves people breathing oxygen at high pressure within special chambers in the same way that deep sea divers are treated for 'the bends'. There is anecdotal evidence that some people with MS find HBO helpful with certain symptoms such as fatigue, visual disturbances and bladder problems. However, clinical trials have failed to confirm HBO as beneficial. Although it appears to be a relatively safe procedure, its routine use cannot be recommended. The centres which use HBO also provide a great deal of information, support and access to other therapies such as physiotherapy and counselling which may be valuable. If you are thinking of trying HBO, it may be helpful to chat with your MS nurse about local availability and costs.

12 | Bladder and bowels

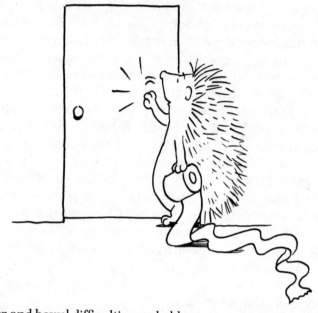

Bladder and bowel difficulties probably cause more inconvenience to people with MS than just about anything else. They can be extremely embarrassing, very difficult to cope with, cause major limitations of your lifestyle, reduce your quality of life and yet can be one of the most difficult problems to discuss with your doctor.

MANAGING BLADDER PROBLEMS

I am very embarrassed about losing control of my bladder and wetting myself on occasions. Is this the result of my MS?

Bladder problems are very common in MS. About 75 per cent (3 out of 4) of people will experience some difficulties at some stage. The sort of symptoms people experience include needing to pass urine more often than usual (urinary frequency), a feeling of needing to pass water urgently (urinary urgency), not being able to pass urine when feeling the urge (urinary hesitancy) and passing water involuntarily leading to 'accidents' (urinary incontinence).

The problems you describe are all too common in MS and experienced by many people, so you are certainly not on your own. The good news is that there is a great deal that can be done to help. The first step is to discuss the problems you are experiencing with your MS nurse, GP or neurologist. You may be need to be referred to a continence adviser – a specialist nurse who works with people who have bladder problems – in order that your difficulties are fully assessed and appropriate treatment options discussed.

I often have to go to the loo very urgently to pass water. It is really embarrassing. Is there anything I can do to control this?

The symptom you are experiencing is called urinary urgency and is very common in MS. Fortunately, a lot can be done to help people suffering from this sort of problem. The most important thing is to discuss this with your MS nurse, GP or neurologist who can then ensure you get the right help.

There are two different ways in which the bladder can stop working properly in MS and while both ways can cause the same symptoms, the treatments are different so it is important that you are properly assessed. The bladder can either become over-sensitive, so that it causes you to want to void when it is only partially full, resulting in urgency and frequency, or it can become under-active, so it may not empty fully and again cause urgency and frequency.

Think of the bladder as a sink with water in it (see Figure 12.1 for two different scenarios). The sink on the left is almost empty containing just a small amount of water. However, if your bladder muscle isn't working properly (detrusor instability), the result can be as if someone is pulling on the plug chain to empty the sink – you will have an urge to pass water. This condition can respond to anticholinergic drugs.

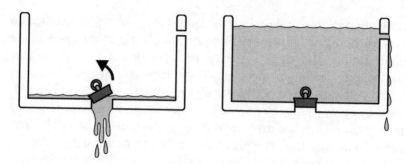

Figure 12.1 Two ways in which your bladder can cause you to have the urge to pass water

The sink on the right is almost full but the plug will not let the water out. Any further water dripping into the sink will result in water passing into the overflow. This has the potential to cause the urge to pass water again. Giving *anticholinergic drugs* in this situation will only make the situation worse by causing further accumulation of water (urine).

For this reason, it is important to differentiate between the two causes of urinary urgency. The best method of doing this is with a bladder scan and this is usually done by a continence adviser. The bladder scan, which is painless, is an ultrasound scan of your bladder taken before and after you have passed urine so that the amount of urine left in your bladder can be calculated. This is crucial as it tells us which of the two 'sink' scenarios we are dealing with either before or after anticholinergic treatment.

The magic number for residual urinary volume is usually 100 ml – approximately one third of a can of cola. If there is more than 100 ml in your bladder after you have passed water, this suggests that you have a bladder that has problems emptying completely and is behaving like the sink on the right. If you have 100 ml or more in your bladder after passing urine, you will be at risk of getting urine infections. Such infections don't just make you feel bad, they can also cause a temporary worsening of your MS symptoms – a 'pseudo-relapse'. The way to treat this problem is to use a small, disposable catheter inserted into the bladder once or more daily to drain off excess urine. This can go a long way towards resolving your symptoms as well as reducing the risk of urine infections. While the thought of using one of these catheters can be very daunting, people who actually use them find it much more straightforward than they had feared and that it makes a huge difference to their quality of life.

If your bladder is found to be emptying fully but is over-sensitive, there are drug treatments (such as the anticholinergic medications including oxybutynin, tolterodine and trospium chloride) which can be used to help stabilise the bladder and ease your symptoms. DDAVP (desmopressin), which is available either as tablets or a nasal spray, can also be helpful if you have to get up frequently during the night or need to go on a long journey where access to toilet facilities may be difficult. This is an anti-diuretic hormone that temporarily stops your kidneys producing urine so your bladder doesn't fill. It can only be used once a day and you will need to discuss this with your doctor in order to ensure it is safe for you to use.

It is important to talk to your MS nurse or continence adviser if you have any queries or concerns about your bladder function. They will be able to set your mind at rest and explain the best course of action in more detail.

I have decided to drink as little as I can because I have so many problems with my bladder. It seems to help. Is this a good idea?

Many people who find they have to go to the toilet more often than usual try and reduce this problem by not drinking very much. This is not a good idea! It is really important to keep drinking as you can make yourself very ill if you become too dehydrated and you may also increase your risk of a urine infection. The more you can drink the more likely you are to be able to flush out any bugs which could otherwise cause an infection. You should aim to drink at least 1 ½ litres (2 ½ pints) of fluid each day. This includes drinks, soup, sauces, milk on cereal, etc. You may also find it helps to change the type of drinks you take. Those with high levels of caffeine such as tea, coffee or cola, can irritate the bladder and cause you to go to the toilet more often.

Fizzy drinks can have the same effect. If you are able to replace caffeine-containing and fizzy drinks with something else you may feel the benefit. If you really feel that you need some caffeine to get going in the morning, have your tea or coffee but see if you can cut down later in the day – try decaffeinated tea or coffee, herbal teas, fruit juices, cordials or still water as alternatives. Don't forget that if you are still having problems you should discuss these with your GP, MS nurse or neurologist as they may be able to suggest other things that might help.

I have two sorts of difficulties with my water works. One is that I can't easily start urinating even though I want to go, and the other is that I still have a feeling that my bladder is relatively full even after I have been. Can I do anything about these problems?

These are very common problems in MS so you are not alone. Even though you feel that you really want to empty your bladder, nothing happens and this can be really frustrating – not to mention inconvenient. Pressing on the bladder area, in the centre of your abdomen below your navel, or standing up, turning round and sitting down again may get you started – this sounds silly but it can help and no one can see you in the loo. Your continence adviser will be able to suggest where you might be able to buy a bladder stimulator (a simple, hand held massage device) which can sometimes help. The feeling you can't empty your bladder properly is also very common. Try the same techniques described for getting started and this may get you going again.

If you are suffering from either of these problems, it is very important to talk to your MS nurse or continence adviser. The continence adviser can assess how much urine is left in your bladder and then talk to you about different treatment options. Your continence nurse may suggest you try self-catheterisation. This may alarm you, but do try not to worry. The process is much more straightforward than it sounds and quite simple to do once you have been shown. It can make a huge difference and give you up to several hours between trips to the toilet.

Will my urinary problems ever get better?

This is a difficult question to answer because everyone with MS is so different. Sometimes MS symptoms, including urinary problems, can flare up and then they settle down again after a while; at other times symptoms may develop more gradually and persist. What is important to realise is that whatever your symptoms, there is something which can be done to help and it is always worth discussing any problems or concerns you may be having with your MS nurse, neurologist or GP. It is worth mentioning that if your urinary symptoms suddenly get worse it may be a sign of an infection, particularly if you have a temperature or develop a burning pain when passing water. If you think you may have an infection, you should visit your GP as soon as possible.

I am taking medication for bladder problems. Should I take it all the time, or can I stop and start when I feel I need to?

Bladder problems tend to be quite persistent once they develop, so it is important to take any prescribed medications on a regular basis to ensure you get the most benefit from them. If you feel that your bladder symptoms may have settled on their own, and you want to see if you can manage without medication, discuss this with whoever prescribed the treatment. They may well agree that stopping medication is appropriate.

PROBLEMS WITH THE BOWELS

I always seem to be constipated. Is this a symptom of the MS or something else?

People with MS often have problems with their bowels and constipation is probably the most common symptom. The muscles in the gut that normally help to move stool through at a reasonable speed to ensure regularity can become weak and this can lead to constipation. It is important to make sure you are drinking plenty and eating a varied diet rich in fruit, vegetables and other fibre. If you keep as active as possible, this will also help. Some people continue to have problems despite doing everything they can to help themselves. In such cases, something extra such as a laxative may be needed. If you are thinking of taking laxatives, you should discuss this first with your GP, MS nurse or pharmacist.

I know about the problems people with MS can have with their bladder – I have some myself – but I have recently been having some bowel problems too. Do people with MS get 'bowel incontinence' like some get 'urinary incontinence'?

Yes. People with MS can sometimes experience bowel incontinence which is obviously very distressing. It can happen when either the bowel muscles get too weak to hold the stool until you can get to the toilet, or if the bowel muscles go into spasm. Bowel incontinence is more difficult to manage than urinary incontinence, but help is still available and you should discuss these problems with your MS nurse, district nurse or GP.

There are a number of different approaches to bowel management which can be helpful. In the first instance it is important to look at your diet and fluid intake. Try keeping a food diary for a couple of weeks to see if there is any particular type of food or drink which seems to be linked to episodes of incontinence and then see if it helps when you avoid that. Monitor as well the amount of fibre that you eat, as too much can also aggravate your symptoms.

It is also important to try to get your bowels into a good routine. Using the gastrocolic reflex can help. This is a reflex which means your bowels are more likely to be active after a meal, especially in the morning. Try to get into the habit of going to the toilet to try and open your bowels each morning after your breakfast, but don't sit and strain for too long. It helps if you can sit on the toilet in a position that makes defecation easier too (see Figure 12.2). If you are able to get

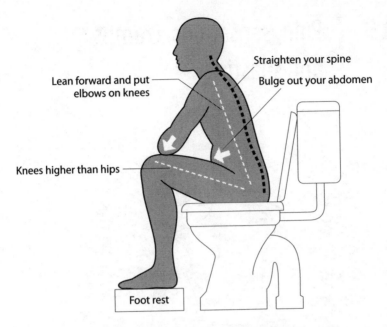

Straighten your spine

Bulge out your abdomen

Lean forward and put elbows on knees

Knees higher than hips

Foot rest

Figure 12.2 The best position for successful defecation

into a good routine of emptying your bowels most mornings, you will be much less likely to experience episodes of incontinence.

If you experience soiling on a regular basis, there is something known as an anal plug which you place just inside your anus and which prevents any soiling. This may sound a little daunting, but it can actually be very helpful. Your GP can prescribe an anal plug for you if he or she thinks one might be useful.

These measures alone may not be enough to manage the problem. If this is the case, your medication may need to be adjusted to help improve control. Taking a combination of a low dose of a medication to constipate you (loperamide syrup is very useful as this can be *titrated* easily and taken in small doses) and a laxative which will help you empty your bowels at a time convenient to you can be effective. Your GP, district nurse or continence adviser will work with you to find the best regimen for you.

13 | Pain, sensations, cramps and spasticity

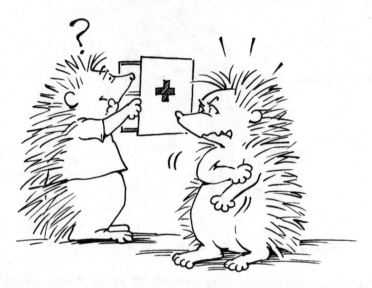

Abnormal sensations, which can seem unusual, deeply unpleasant and painful are unfortunately not uncommon symptoms of MS. Standard painkillers do not work for pain caused by nerve damage. Spasticity and spasms also reflect the consequences of nerve damage. In this chapter we explain all of these symptoms and how they are best managed both by medication and other means.

Following my diagnosis with MS, I have started experiencing some pain and tightness in my chest. Climbing stairs can really wind me. Should I bother my doctor, and what can be done about it?

It is very important to understand that you, just like anyone else, can become ill from conditions other than MS; not every twinge, pain or symptom may be due to MS. What you describe may be nothing serious, but the symptoms are not typical of MS and could be due to angina. You *must* consult your GP. It is important to have an understanding of the type of symptoms typical of MS in order to recognise those that are not and may be due to other causes. If in doubt, discuss any new symptoms with your MS nurse or GP.

NERVE PAIN

I seem to be getting several aches and pains in various parts of my body, but I have been told that MS is not a painful disease. Is this true?

People with MS have known for many years that specific symptoms can cause considerable pain, and this is now being recognised. Chronic pain is experienced by about 50 per cent (1 in 2) of people with MS and almost everyone will experience some kind of pain at some point.

Pain in MS may have a number of causes. It may be directly related to MS nerve damage (neuropathic pain), occur as a result of muscular weakness and its complications (nocioceptive pain) or be a mixture of the two. Non-nerve pain caused by muscular weakness can predispose to poor posture and abnormal walking patterns, which themselves can place undue stresses and strains on your muscles, ligaments and joints, causing pain. Prevention is better than cure in this respect. An up-to-date physiotherapy assessment if your walking is a problem, or a wheelchair assessment if you are unable to walk, can be invaluable in reducing problems later on. Non-nerve pain, when present, will usually respond at least temporarily to paracetamol, non-steroidal anti-inflammatory drugs like ibuprofen and diclofenac, and, if really necessary, codeine-based medications.

Pain can also occur as a result of stiffness and spasms. We discuss ways of reducing and managing spasticity later in this chapter. Some doctors consider spasm-related pain to be nerve pain, others do not.

'Pain in an area of numbness' is very characteristic of nerve (neuropathic) pain. After nerves are damaged the normal messages they carry may not get through as well (reduced sensation) or not at all (total numbness). At the same time, various chemical changes occur in damaged nerves with the result that they become much more excitable. This results in a 'double whammy' – pain in an otherwise numb area. The nerves may activate spontaneously, which accounts for spontaneous burning, shooting pains or pins and needles that some people experience. Damaged nerves can also sometimes respond in an exaggerated way to normal stimuli which then feel painful. Examples would include painful irritation in response to the pressure of bedsheets or someone brushing against you or stroking your skin, or certain types of material like lycra against the skin. For some people, hot or cold sensations may feel abnormally painful. This is called *allodynia*. Of course, there can also be a greater appreciation of normally painful stimuli too, as nerves normally lie in insulated bundles adjacent to each other. Once nerve damage occurs and a number of highly excitable nerve endings lie close to each other, you can imagine that they may cross-talk or short circuit each other. This explains spontaneous, sometimes highly unusual, sensations such as the sensation of water trickling down your skin, when it feels bone dry. Other people feel a crawling sensation, as if insects are moving on the skin or more commonly burning, sharp, tight, or sensations *deep down* within the bone, that despite scratching the skin refuse to go away.

What is the commonest form of nerve pain in MS?

The most common form of nerve (or neuropathic) pain in MS is called dysaesthesia. This is an abnormal unpleasant sensation that is often described as burning, pricking or stabbing in nature. It usually affects the lower limbs and may be continuous or intermittent and triggered by movement, exercise or temperature. It can sometimes be more noticeable in the evenings, either as a result of physical activity during the day, or because you are less distracted at the end of the day.

I sometimes feel I have cold water running down my leg and I have to check that it is not wet. At other times my leg burns and sometimes it feels as if someone is stabbing me. Why is this?

When nerves are damaged in MS a number of changes occur within them. The end result is that they can start 'misfiring' for no apparent reason. For example, the nerves that normally send messages to the brain only when the skin is wet, cold or hot may start to send messages spontaneously, inappropriately and without any obvious trigger, so that your brain interprets your skin as being wet, cold or burning when it is not. This process may also cause abnormal dagger-like pains known as *neuralgia*.

What are the common drugs used for nerve pain in MS and how should I take them?

Standard painkillers such as ibuprofen and paracetamol do not work for nerve pain. Opioids such as codeine, dihydrocodeine and even morphine do not tend to relieve nerve pain as well as they do nocioceptive (tissue damage) pain. This leaves so-called 'atypical' painkillers as the options to treat nerve pain.

There are very few licensed drugs in the UK for the treatment of neuropathic (nerve) pain. They include gabapentin (Neurontin) which is given up to three times daily and a very similar drug called pregabalin (Lyrica) which is given twice daily. These are both drugs that are used to treat epilepsy, and they raise the threshold at which the nerves activate to carry messages and so reduce their irritability. Carbamazepine (Tegretol) and phenytoin (Epanutin) are two other anti-epilepsy drugs which are licensed for the treatment of trigeminal neuralgia, but are sometimes used for other types of nerve pain too including burning dysaesthetic pain in the limbs. The other major class of drugs which are sometimes helpful are certain types of antidepressants, especially those called *tricyclics* such as amitriptyline and nortriptyline. In other nerve pain conditions other classes of antidepressants called SNRIs such as duloxetine (Cymbalta) are also effective although there is no published evidence of this in MS as yet.

Whichever medication your neurologist prescribes for your nerve pain, there are a few common pieces of advice. Drugs for nerve pain are started at a deliberately low dose to avoid side effects. Therefore it is possible that the first few doses may not cause any effects, good or bad, and this means that you should ask your GP or MS nurse how to increase the medication or follow any *titration* schedule that you have been given until you get an effect. If you get minor side effects they can settle if you remain on the current dose of medication for a week or two longer. Typical daily start doses for commonly used drugs for nerve pain would be: gabapentin 100 mg to 300 mg; pregabalin 50 mg to 75 mg (we find this is better tolerated in people with MS than the 150 mg suggested in the product literature), carbamazepine 100 mg to 200 mg (the Retard long acting preparation is usually better tolerated). Amitriptyline or nortriptyline can be started at between 10 mg and 25 mg at night as they can cause drowsiness and you can use this to your advantage to promote a good night's sleep. The other drugs for nerve pain are best started at night too, so that you sleep off any side effects while your body gets used to them.

People with MS vary enormously in terms of how well they tolerate drugs for nerve pain. Some people for example will feel 'like a zombie' when taking as little as 5 mg of amitriptyline, whereas other people can take over 100 mg without any good or bad effects whatsoever.

We cannot predict whether an individual person will respond at all to a particular medication or whether they will get side effects. This is why it is important to start slowly and increase slowly, usually at a minimum of weekly to fortnightly intervals. If you are not sure whether you feel 'better', 'the same', or 'worse', stay on the same dose of drug until you can be sure. In this way you will take the smallest effective dose.

My neurologist has prescribed me a medication for nerve pain. When I looked at the information leaflet it did not mention pain, but said that the drug is for epilepsy. I don't have epilepsy, so why am I being prescribed this?

In MS, damaged nerves can become over-sensitive and start 'misfiring' without receiving a trigger to do so. This has some similarities with the process that causes fits (or seizures) in a person with epilepsy and is the reason anti-epilepsy drugs are often helpful in people who have nerve (neuropathic) pain. Don't worry – you don't have epilepsy. Epilepsy is not a common problem in people with MS.

My neurologist has prescribed me a medication for nerve pain. When I looked at the information leaflet it did not mention pain, but that this drug is used for depression. Does the doctor think the pain is 'all in my mind'?

No – your doctor does not think your pain is imaginary or due to depression. An antidepressant drug has been prescribed because it works in a way that may be beneficial for nerve (neuropathic) pain in MS. The old-style tricyclic antidepressant drugs (amitriptyline, nortriptyline, imipramine) are often used for this purpose and usually at much lower doses than required to treat depression.

I have been very worried about the possible side effects of the drug I have been prescribed for nerve pain. The information leaflet that came with the tablets describes side effects that sound just like many of the symptoms I already have from MS. Why is this?

Drugs which help to relieve nerve pain are thought to stop nerves activating inappropriately. Unfortunately sometimes they can slow or stop normal nerve impulses and temporarily cause a number of side effects – such as weakness, numbness and pins and needles – that are similar to symptoms of MS. These symptoms also occur in people without MS who are prescribed these drugs.

It is impossible to say whether or not a particular drug for nerve pain will be helpful, and at what dose, or whether it will cause significant side effects. Therefore starting off at the smallest dose and building the dose up slowly over weeks or months can be a sensible approach, so that you know what effect has been achieved, before you increase the dose further. If you do experience side effects, they will often settle down with time as your body becomes accustomed to the medication and staying on the same dose of medication for an extra week or two can help to reduce side effects as can increasing the drug by a smaller dose. Sometimes, if you are taking amitriptylene or a similar drug, chewing sugar-free chewing gum can help to reduce dryness in the mouth by stimulating production of saliva.

My neurologist prescribed me a drug for nerve pain. I took it for a couple of weeks but it didn't work, so I stopped taking it. Why didn't it work and what should I do?

It is very likely you did not take enough of the drug. Your neurologist will have purposefully started you on a very low dose in order to minimise side effects. It is not surprising, therefore, that you did not feel any benefit over such a short period of time. You will need to restart the medication and slowly build up the dose until you either get sufficient pain relief or experience troublesome side effects. If it is helpful and well tolerated it should be continued, but otherwise you should stop treatment. Your neurologist will be able to advise on other treatment options.

How quickly should I increase the drug I have been prescribed for nerve pain?

The simple answer is to take as long as you need to decide whether the current dose of the drug you are taking is making you feel better, worse or is having no effect. It generally takes a week or so to allow most of the drugs discussed in this chapter to reach a steady level in your bloodstream. If it is not having any beneficial effect, you may not be taking enough and you will need to increase the dose. If you are experiencing troublesome side effects this may not be an option and you will need to consider reducing the dose and stopping treatment. Your doctor may then prescribe a different drug to be tried in the same way.

Is it possible that my nerve pain will be cured or go away by itself?

The drug treatments for nerve pain usually take the edge off the pain rather than stopping it completely. It is important to have realistic expectations in order to avoid disappointment. Encouragingly, some people find that even small reductions in pain severity can make a big difference to their quality of life. Although it is always possible your pain may go away by itself at any time, the longer you have had the pain, the less likely this is to happen.

Is long-term pain related to other symptoms in MS?

Yes. Pain can have an adverse effect on your sleep pattern, contribute to low mood and increase fatigue. On the other hand if your pain is treated successfully, you may find your sleep pattern, mood and fatigue also improve. These added benefits might, in turn, help you cope better with any other problems you may have due to your condition.

ALTERED SENSATIONS

I sometimes get pins and needles and occasionally a burning sensation in my legs. What is happening?

These symptoms are very likely to be due to MS. The sensation of pins and needles and burning occurs due to abnormal nerve signals being received by the brain from particular areas of your body.

Typically, these symptoms may get worse at night or following exercise. Some people take tricyclic antidepressant, drugs, anti-epilepsy drugs or opiate (codeine and morphine-derived) drugs if the sensations are troublesome. If tablet treatments are inadequate, sometimes additional measures such as transcutaneous electrical nerve stimulation (TENS) can be helpful. This is a technique where a tiny electric current is applied to the area concerned by a small portable machine. Your doctor will be able to discuss these therapeutic options.

I have had a feeling of numbness quite frequently in my left arm, and then the other day on the right side of my face. Can I do anything about this?

Numbness, a term usually used to describe a lack of sensation, is quite a common symptom in MS and is due to an inability of your nerves to send signals from a particular part of your body to your brain. Any part of your body can be affected in this way. Numbness in the hands can make it difficult for you to feel, hold and pick things up, whereas numbness in your legs can cause unsteadiness. Although drugs can help symptoms such as pins and needles and pain caused by oversensitive nerves, these sorts of treatments do not usually help symptoms such as numbness. You may find you have to rely more on your other senses, and vision in particular, to compensate for this lack of sensation.

I find hot days are a big problem. Not only does my MS get worse, but I also get a lot of pain. Why is this?

People with MS often find heat is a problem. This is due to the nerves not being able to work properly in hot conditions or with vigorous exercise. You may find that you experience temporary fatigue, blurred vision, numbness, pain or weakness at these times and that these symptoms improve once you have cooled down. This is a characteristic feature of MS known as *Uhthoff's phenomenon*, named after the German ophthalmologist who first described it. You may need to alter your lifestyle – for example, by avoiding vigorous exercise or exposure to hot temperatures – in order to minimise the impact this problem has on your day-to-day activities.

Each time I bend my neck forward I get an odd electric shock sensation down my back and arms. What is this and what causes it?

You are describing *Lhermitte's phenomenon*, named after the French neurologist who first published a report describing it. It is also known as the Barber Chair phenomenon for obvious reasons. The people who experience this symptom usually describe a brief sensation of electricity or tingling that travels down from their neck to the lower back or limbs, when their chin is placed upon the chest. It is caused by the temporary stretching and irritation of damaged nerves in the back of the spinal cord at neck level. Curiously, people often do not tell their doctor about this problem because it is so unusual and they may not think it is relevant. If a young adult person develops Lhermitte's phenomenon, this is highly suggestive of MS. However, there are other causes of Lhermitte's phenomenon, including vitamin B12 deficiency. In older people it is often due to 'wear and tear' or a slipped disc in the neck causing pressure on the nerves.

Recently I had excruciating brief sharp stabs of pain in my cheek. I couldn't eat anything, shave or even touch my face. What was this?

It sounds as if you are describing a condition called trigeminal neuralgia. People often describe trigeminal neuralgia as the worst pain they have ever experienced. The trigeminal nerve is so called as it splits into three to supply the skin of the face; the forehead above the eyebrow, the cheek area and the jaw. Neuralgia refers to nerve pain which is brief, electric-shock like and sharp or stabbing. A lot of people describe it as being like having a sharp object stuck into their face. Trigeminal neuralgia usually affects the cheek or jaw area and can be confused with other conditions, for example dental disease. It is triggered by usually innocuous stimuli such as talking, eating, brushing teeth, shaving or touching the face especially the central area at the base of the nose, the top or bottom lips. The pain of trigeminal neuralgia may also occur spontaneously without any trigger.

In people without MS, the usual cause of trigeminal neuralgia is pressure on the nerve by a blood vessel which causes wearing away of the myelin insulation at that point of the nerve, causing it to be more excitable and to activate with little or no trigger. In MS, where trigeminal neuralgia is 20 times more common than in the general population, it tends to occur at a younger age and can occur on both sides of the face. The cause is usually inflammatory demyelination of the trigeminal nerve, just as can occur in other parts of the brain and spinal cord. Of course, people with MS could occasionally have trigeminal neuralgia because of a blood vessel pressing on a nerve, and your neurologist will consider performing an MRI scan to rule this out.

What are the treatment options for trigeminal neuralgia?

The mainstay of drug treatment for trigeminal neuralgia is carbamazepine (Tegretol), and steroid therapy for the inflammation. Carbamazepine is often very effective, and is used to treat the pain of trigeminal neuralgia in people with and without MS. If someone with MS has developed trigeminal neuralgia within the last few weeks, high dose steroids may be used – as they could for any relapse – to reduce inflammation in and around the nerve. Alternatives to carbamazepine include phenytion (Epanutin), gabapentin (Neurontin), pregabalin (Lyrica) and baclofen (Lioresal). Whichever drug you take, as with other forms of neuropathic pain, you will need to increase the dose you take over time until you reach a dose that is helpful without causing limiting side effects.

Other non-drug treatments for trigeminal neuralgia do not seem to be as effective for people with MS as for those without MS, probably because the causes are different as described above. However, as these non-drug techniques are occasionally used for people with MS, it is worth discussing them. There are essentially four groups of techniques which target the trigeminal nerve progressively more deeply:

- The first set of techniques involves the injection of substances, or the use of heat, to either block or destroy the trigeminal nerve.

- The second group of techniques involves the passage of a needle into the skull through a naturally occurring hole (the foramen ovale) and then selected destruction or damage of part of the nerve via thermal, chemical or mechanical techniques, the latter involving a balloon which compresses the nerve.

- The next option involves targeted radiotherapy to a specific deep area of the trigeminal nerve.

- Finally, an open neurosurgical operation called a microvascular decompression is the most radical, but some would argue in carefully selected cases, the most successful treatment.

A recent expert review concluded that there was insufficient evidence to recommend any specific surgical procedure for people with MS and trigeminal neuralgia. Therefore, the options you are offered by your neurosurgeon will depend upon your general health, other medical conditions, whether or not you have a blood vessel pressing on the trigeminal nerve and what risks you are prepared to accept for the potential success of each procedure. You should weigh up these issues carefully after a full and frank discussion with your neurosurgeon.

CRAMPS AND SPASTICITY

I often get what seem to be cramps or spasms in my legs. They often go rigid, the cramps are very painful and they are making my life really difficult. What can I do?

What you are describing is known as spasticity. This is due to damage to the nerve pathways that travel from your brain, along the spinal cord to the muscles in your trunk, arms and legs. The nerves can become oversensitive and misfire, causing stiffness, cramps and painful spasms due to several muscles contracting simultaneously. People who develop spasticity often find their legs may be weak and that they also have some walking difficulties and bladder problems. Spasticity is a common problem in MS and it usually affects muscles in the calf, thigh or buttock areas, as well as the lower back and, occasionally, the arms. It is important you seek help because, if it is not treated at an early stage, spasticity can eventually lead to contractures, where the muscle and tendons shorten, causing more pain and making it impossible for you to straighten your limbs properly.

Regular exercise, such as swimming, is one of the best ways of managing this problem at an early stage. Stretching exercises and input from a physiotherapist may also be very helpful. If these measures are inadequate, drug treatments may also be considered. One of the most widely used and effective drugs is baclofen (Lioresal). Other muscle relaxants include dantrolene (Dantrium) and tizanidine (Zanaflex).

I think something is happening to my left foot – it's no longer as straight as it was and it seems to have 'turned in'. What can I do?

This can happen sometimes and is a result of muscles on one side of your foot shortening more than on the other side, which can happen for a variety of reasons. Don't worry, though, as something can be done. Contact the local physiotherapists for advice – if you don't have a contact number for them ask your MS nurse, GP or neurologist as they can refer you to the local neuro-rehabilitation team. The physiotherapists will then assess the problem and suggest exercises which can help. They may also discuss with you other treatment options depending on the severity of the problem.

I have had MS for a number of years and I now cannot walk. My worst symptom is that my legs are so stiff I cannot bend them and often they go into spasm. I am taking tablets but they don't seem to be working. Is there anything else that can be done?

Unfortunately, some people go on to get severe spasticity despite all the standard treatments being used. If severe spasticity develops in someone who uses a walking aid or wheelchair, it is very important to pay close attention to stretch exercises, posture, seating position, avoidance of pressure sores and the early identification and prompt treatment of bladder infections. Very occasionally, treatment with intra-thecal baclofen may be considered – this involves the continuous infusion of a tiny amount of muscle relaxant directly into the space around the spinal cord in the lower back via a small pump. This sort of treatment is only available in a few specialist centres. If you develop contractures despite all these measures, surgery to lengthen the tendons that connect the muscles to bone may be considered.

14 | Fatigue, cognition and mood

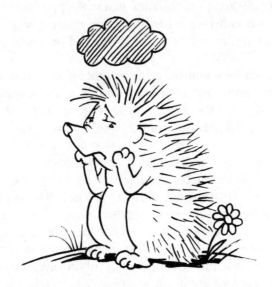

Fatigue or tiredness is one of the most debilitating symptoms of MS, and one that worries many people. Some ideas for managing fatigue are given in the first half of this chapter. People with MS may also develop problems with their memory, thinking and mood – these important, but often neglected, problems are considered in the later part of the chapter.

FATIGUE

The worst symptom of my MS seems to be fatigue. I feel I can hardly do anything. Not only that, it seems to come when I least expect it. What causes it?

Fatigue is a symptom experienced by the majority of people with MS at some time. Both the ability to carry out physical activities, and the ability to concentrate or think, may be affected. It can affect people who have only mild or no disability and it does not seem to be directly related to depression.

Although fatigue in MS is poorly understood, there are a number of important factors that contribute. Nerves that have lost their myelin insulation may be able to function normally until they have to work too hard and become exhausted. The immune system may release chemicals that cause a feeling of fatigue and people with MS may need to use more parts of their brain to achieve the same result as someone who does not have MS, because of damage to some of the nerve pathways. A combination of all these different mechanisms may be responsible for fatigue in MS.

I seem to suffer badly with fatigue. Is there anything I can do to help myself?

The management of fatigue is difficult and reliably effective medication is not currently available. A practical approach can sometimes be helpful. Fatigue is often worst in the afternoon, perhaps because body temperature is naturally higher at this time. Structuring the day so that less activity is required at this time may therefore be beneficial. Unfortunately, this option isn't open to everyone. It is also a good idea to give yourself sufficient time to recover from each task during the day, rather than rushing from one activity to the next. A good night's sleep is also important. Bladder problems and pain may interrupt sleep – improving these symptoms may mean you are less tired during the day.

There is some evidence from clinical trials that a drug called amantadine (Symmetrel) may help fatigue in some people with MS. Unfortunately, this treatment is beneficial in a minority of people only. Another drug called modafinil (Provigil) can reduce daytime sleepiness but probably doesn't help fatigue in any other regard. Because daytime sleepiness is a problem that doesn't affect many people with MS in a major way, this treatment is not usually particularly effective. Exercise programmes, or other structured physical activities such as yoga or pilates, do seem to help the symptoms of fatigue in some people with MS.

What is the difference between fatigue and laziness?

Fatigue is a feeling of tiredness and exhaustion, often associated with a reduced capacity to carry out mental and physical activities over which you have no voluntary control. The term laziness, in contrast, is usually used to describe a mental attitude characterised by inertia, apathy and lack of voluntary effort that you can wilfully overcome. If you are suffering from MS-related fatigue, you are not lazy!

Following exercise, my symptoms are worse for a few hours. Should I exercise or not?

Exercise can cause temporary worsening of symptoms in people with MS in three major ways:

1. Most people will notice it takes a little time to recover following exercise. A person with MS may notice this more. For example, they may experience increasing heaviness of their legs and ultimately may need to stop and rest if they have similar, but milder, problems before they begin to exercise. This sort of problem is probably just an exaggeration of the normal effects of exercise on our body.

2. Small increases in body temperature can reduce the ability of damaged nerves that have lost their myelin to work properly. As a result, when some people with MS exercise, have a fever or take a hot bath, they can sometimes experience a temporary worsening or recurrence of previous symptoms. This is called *Uhthoff's phenomenon* or the 'hot bath effect'. A relatively common example of this is a brief reduction in the vision in one eye previously affected by inflammation of the optic nerve (optic neuritis). No new damage is being done

when this happens, so it is not harmful to carry on exercising if it is comfortable to do so.

❸ Fatigue can make exercising difficult and can itself be worsened by physical exertion. However, if exercise is done in manageable amounts and there is time to recover afterwards, overall levels of fatigue may actually be reduced in the medium and long-term. It is generally thought that exercise is good for MS, as it is for most people. Most health professionals would therefore recommend regular exercise that can be done comfortably, does not involve heavy weights, does not lead to exhaustion and following which there is adequate time for recovery before it is repeated.

In summary, do small amounts often and exercise within your limits!

COGNITIVE AND MENTAL PROBLEMS

I thought MS is a disease of the body and your mind isn't affected at all. Am I wrong?

Yes and no – it depends what you mean by the words 'body' and 'mind'. When most people talk about a problem with the 'body' they are usually referring to physical difficulties such as weakness, numbness or clumsiness, whereas when they talk of problems with the 'mind' they usually mean cognitive or mental difficulties such as poor memory or low mood. Because MS affects the brain, and the brain controls both the 'body' and the 'mind', it can cause all of these problems. That said, as a general rule, physical difficulties are usually very obvious, whereas cognitive and mental problems are easily missed, overlooked or ignored. It is for this reason that cognitive and mental difficulties are considered as potentially 'hidden' problems in MS. Healthcare professionals need to look actively for these hidden symptoms so that they can be identified and treated.

What are cognitive problems?

Cognition is a term that is used to describe our ability to do a wide variety of tasks such as communicate, recognise things, remember, learn and plan. It was thought until recently that memory problems and some other cognitive difficulties were a rare occurrence in MS. However, more recent research has shown that a wide range of cognitive problems, varying both in nature and severity, may be present in many people with MS.

Why is cognition affected in MS?

The brain may be considered as a complex network of nerves (neurons) that are linked and communicate with each other and with parts of the body. MS is a condition that causes patches of inflammation and nerve damage throughout the brain – this can disrupt and slow down these communications and thereby reduce how well the brain can function. All this can result in problems with cognition that usually manifests as an overall slowing of cognitive abilities and particular problems with memory and thinking.

How will I know whether I have cognitive problems?

Cognitive problems in MS usually present themselves as difficulties with memory and thinking – they may be very subtle and easily missed. Indeed, it may be family, friends or work colleagues that first notice something is wrong rather than the person affected. You may notice difficulty with day-to-day memory such as remembering recent events or important things you need to do. You may find your powers of concentration are reduced and that you have difficulty planning, learning new tasks, doing complex things or doing more than one thing at the same time. Some people also notice word finding difficulties and that their thought processes are generally slowed down or seem to be more effortful. All of these difficulties may be exacerbated by fatigue, low mood, anxiety and stress. If you have any concerns, it is important to share them and seek advice from your neurologist, MS nurse or GP, particularly if the difficulties are having a significant impact on your day-to-day life.

Will my cognitive problems get worse?

This is very difficult to predict. It is entirely possible that your problems will remain unchanged for many years or temporarily improve or worsen due to fatigue, low mood, anxiety or stress. Although it is true that some people with MS go on to develop quite severe cognitive problems (dementia) over many years, most do not. Encouragingly, there are many things you can do to help to reduce the impact any cognitive difficulties are having on your day-to-day activities and improve your quality of life. This is discussed in more detail later in this chapter.

Are there any drugs that I can take to help my memory?

At present, there aren't any drugs you can take to improve your cognitive abilities. However, it is seems likely that new drug treatments will be available in the future. For now it is important to appreciate that some existing drug treatments used in MS may actually have an adverse effect on your cognition. It is therefore important to check the drugs you are currently taking with your GP, neurologist or MS nurse because stopping one or more of them may be helpful. Your cognitive abilities may be also be impaired if you are low in mood – if this is the case, medication for depression may be beneficial. Encouragingly, clinical trials have shown that early treatment with disease-modifying drugs may reduce the long-term accumulation of cognitive problems over time but this is not fully known.

In addition to all these considerations, there are plenty of other things you can do to minimise any cognitive problems and the impact they have on your day-to-day life. These are discussed in more detail in the following answer.

I think my memory is going and I am having problems concentrating. If there are no drugs to help what can I do?

There are plenty of things you can do to improve your concentration and minimise your memory problems. If your powers of concentration are reduced, you may find difficulty planning, learning new tasks, doing complex things or doing more than one thing at once. If you can reduce the number of distractions (for example, turn off your radio or television and divert your telephone), break complex tasks into smaller parts and only do one thing at a time, you may find you can achieve more in your day-to-day activities. It is also worthwhile trying to do things when you feel at your best and avoid trying to do too much when you are feeling tired or fatigued – pace yourself and take rests if possible. It may be helpful to give yourself more time than usual to achieve things in order to avoid frustration and putting yourself under unnecessary pressure. If you have particular problems with your memory, using a calendar, diary or electronic organiser will help you to remind yourself of important information such as telephone numbers, shopping lists and appointments. If you use a calendar, make sure it is displayed in a prominent place and always keep your diary or electronic organiser in the same place where you can find it easily. It is often helpful to establish routines and encourage family, friends and work colleagues to try and fit in with these. If other people are made aware of your difficulties, and the reason you have problems, it is much more likely they will be helpful and supportive. Although this advice may seem like common sense, it can often make a big difference and help you cope better both at home and at work.

My husband sometimes 'loses the plot' when he is speaking to people. We both find it difficult to deal with this – is there anything we can do?

Your husband's cognitive problems may have an impact on other people including family, friends and work colleagues. If they do not understand the nature of his problems, it is easy for others to misinterpret his difficulties and this can make the whole situation worse. It may be helpful for acquaintances to be informed of your husband's problems in order that they can make allowances. If others know he needs more time to answer or to do things, it may reduce the risk of them getting frustrated or misinterpreting your husband's difficulties as being due to lack of interest or laziness. When you are with your husband, he may prefer you to answer on his behalf or to prompt him if he forgets something. These common sense considerations can make a big difference.

Do people with MS suffer from dementia?

Dementia is simply a term used to describe a severe form of cognitive impairment. It can have a number of different causes, the most common of which is Alzheimer's disease. It is important not to use the term inappropriately because this can be misleading and may cause considerable alarm and distress.

Although it is true MS can cause cognitive impairment, this is usually relatively mild and not severe enough to be diagnosed as dementia. It is uncommon for a person with MS to develop severe cognitive impairment and be diagnosed with dementia. If this does happen, it usually occurs after many years and at a time when the affected person has already accumulated significant physical disability. It is also important to appreciate that MS is not linked to any other conditions that cause dementia, including Alzheimer's disease.

DEPRESSION

Do people with MS suffer from mental illness?

Mental illness is a rather broad, non-specific and often stigma-tising term that is not particularly helpful when used in the context of a condition such as MS. It is important to appreciate that mental illness of one sort or another is very common in the general population – 25 per cent of people (1 in 4) will experience some kind of mental health problem over the course of a year. It is therefore not surprising that people with MS may also develop problems with their mood and emotions, as there is no reason why they are any less likely than anyone else to develop mental health problems. It is very important to identify such problems early because there are treatments and therapies available that may help.

In the remaining questions in this chapter, we look at some mental problems that may be more common in people with MS.

I have heard that depression is very common in MS. Is this the case?

Depression is thought to be about twice as common in people with MS as in the general population. Depression is more likely to be mild than severe, to the extent it may sometimes not have been recognised either by the affected person or their doctor. The treatment of depression in people with MS is no different from that for people who do not have MS, and it is often very helpful. If you have any concerns, you should discuss them with your MS nurse or GP.

Why do people with MS have such a high rate of depression?

There is some evidence to show that depression may be more common in people with MS than those with other unrelated neurological conditions of similar severity. This might mean that depression sometimes results from a direct effect of MS on the brain. For example, MS might increase the risk of depression by altering the levels of chemicals that influence mood, or it might cause damage to a part of the brain that controls mood and emotion. Alternatively, the way MS is perceived by the general population and society as a whole might make affected people more vulnerable. Having said all this, most people with MS who become depressed probably do so as a reaction to their circumstances rather than because of anything specifically to do with MS itself. This so-called reactive depression happens to people with and without MS when there are difficulties in their life or when there is worry about the future.

I really can't think of the future at all and I just seem to be living for the present. My wife says that I have dreadful mood swings and I know this upsets her. Is it my MS?

People with MS do seem to have mood swings more than other people. A rare and extreme example of this is bipolar affective disorder – sometimes called 'manic depression'. This causes periods of severe depression (or 'lows') that alternate with periods of uncontrolled mania (or 'highs'). Although this condition is more common in people with MS than in the general population, it is still very rare. Most people with MS who have mood swings will never develop any kind of severe psychiatric illness like bipolar affective disorder. As with depression, it is likely that mood swings happen because of the person's reaction to having MS. Having said that, mood swings can sometimes be due to the direct effect MS can have on parts of the brain that control mood. Standard treatment approaches including counselling, cognitive behavioural therapy or anti-depressant medication may be needed – it is important to discuss these therapeutic options with your MS nurse or GP.

I am worried that I seem to break into tears very easily, or laugh almost uncontrollably at times. My husband is very concerned, as indeed am I. Is there anything I can do about this?

Some people with MS can suffer from a tendency to cry or laugh uncontrollably. Often the crying or the laughter will not be accompanied by the usual associated emotions of sadness or joy. This sort of problem is also seen in other neurological conditions unrelated to MS, and particularly in those which cause damage to the front parts of the brain. This is because the forebrain is responsible for controlling the level and expression of our emotions. Although antidepressants are sometimes tried in this situation, the results are often disappointing. Fortunately, it is rare for uncontrolled laughter and crying to be a persistent and severe problem, and most people adjust well to this in the long-term.

15 | Mobility (including driving), balance and tremor

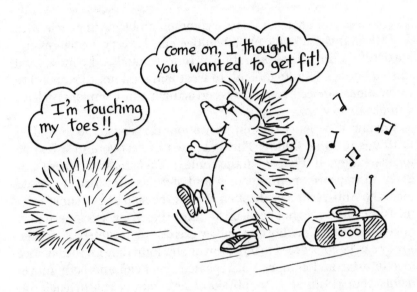

Poor mobility or difficulty getting around is perhaps one of the symptoms people most associate with MS and is often cited as one of the most difficult problems people living with MS have to deal with. Here, we look at some of the symptoms which can cause problems with mobility here and discuss some of the ways these can be eased.

In this chapter we also look at the impact problems with mobility can have on day-to-day living and suggest ways in which getting around can be made easier as well as looking at different things you can do to help yourself stay as strong as possible.

BALANCE

I sometimes feel dizzy and have, on occasions, lost my balance. I don't want people to think I am drunk. Can I do anything about it?

Dizziness and unsteadiness are common problems in people with MS and these sorts of difficulties can be very embarrassing particularly in social situations. Unfortunately, dizziness and unsteadiness are quite difficult to treat and tend not to respond to medications – indeed, some drugs can actually cause similar problems or make them worse.

You may experience spinning sensations that cause you to hold on to things to avoid falling. This is known as vertigo and it can be incapacitating. If it occurs in the context of a *brainstem* relapse, it is likely to improve spontaneously and steroids may help to speed recovery. Anti-vertigo medication can also be helpful as a short-term measure but should not be taken for more than a few weeks as it may impede recovery. Cawthorne-Cooksey exercises can often be beneficial – they can be considered to be a form of physiotherapy for the balance mechanisms and comprise of repeated eye, head and body movements. Your MS nurse, GP or physiotherapist may be able to teach you how to do these.

If you are very unsteady on your feet it is a good idea to consider walking aids – the use of a stick or crutch may reduce the risk of you falling and injuring yourself. At the very least, using such aids will indicate to others that you are not drunk, but that you have a physical problem with balance.

Can you train yourself to wear high heels again?

This depends on your individual circumstances. Some people with MS are able to wear high heels most of the time, and only have to resort to flat shoes at the time of a relapse. However, most people with MS find wearing heels very difficult – balance becomes much more of a problem because there is only a small area to support your weight. You also need to have sufficient strength in your leg muscles and any lack of sensation in your feet may also complicate matters. Wearing high heels can also cause spasm and pain. If you are particularly keen to get back into high heels, we suggest that you first discuss this with your physiotherapist or MS nurse who can give you advice specific to your circumstances.

EXERCISES

Are there any exercises I can do that may help my walking difficulties?

Regular exercise can be very beneficial to your general health. It can also help specific difficulties you may have with walking by keeping the leg muscles and those that help with posture in good working order, and strengthening those that have become weak. Exercise can help reduce spasticity and keep your joints mobile and prevent them from getting stiff. These improvements may, in turn, help with your balance and coordination.

If you have walking difficulties, ask to be referred to a physiotherapist for a mobility assessment. This will provide insights into your posture, the way you walk and the sorts of things you can do to improve your mobility: walking aids may be recommended. Your physiotherapist will be able to show you how to do any exercises that are needed and how to use walking aids properly. Regrettably, your physiotherapist may only be able to spend about an hour a week for a few weeks treating you. It is important, therefore, that you keep up with the specific exercises recommended in between therapy sessions, and after they have ended, in order to get the most benefit and maintain any improvements you have gained.

Private physiotherapy may be an option for some, though this can be costly. If you wish to pursue this further, check with your local MS Society and/or MS Therapy Centre as they may be able to recommend someone and in some instances may be able to help with the costs. It is also important to check that the private physiotherapist has specialist training in neurology and has worked with people with MS previously. All professionals should be happy to tell you about their qualifications and training if you ask.

I have difficulty getting around my house and walking outside. What professional help is available?

If you are having any difficulty walking or getting around, there is a lot of help available. Physiotherapists are experts at helping people improve their mobility. You may need to ask your MS nurse, neurologist or GP to refer you to a local physiotherapist or you may be able to do this yourself. It is important that you try to ensure you are referred to a physiotherapist who has been trained to deal with neurological problems and has experience in treating people with MS. This will enable him or her to give you the best possible advice and treatment.

Another professional who may be able to help is an occupational therapist. It is often possible to identify equipment and home adaptations that may be beneficial, such as an extra stair rail to help you get up and down stairs or a perching stool for the kitchen so you can sit while preparing meals, for example. Occupational therapists can usually be contacted either directly or via your physiotherapist, MS nurse or GP.

How will a physiotherapist evaluate my problems of movement and balance?

At your first appointment, your physiotherapist will want to make sure he or she has all the necessary information about your MS and how it affects you. The physiotherapist will also want to know about the particular problems you are experiencing and what you need help with. He or she will then need to look at the way you move, assess your balance, determine whether you can get up and down stairs, and how well you are able to get in and out of a chair, and so on. The assessment will be tailored to your abilities and the nature of the problems you are experiencing.

Once the assessment has been completed, and the physiotherapist has discussed with you the goals you want to achieve, you will be given exercises that are specific to you and your needs, and designed to help you achieve these goals. As the physiotherapist can usually only see you about once a week for a few weeks, it is very important that you make the most of these sessions and do your best to complete the exercises. This will help you achieve your goals more quickly.

Table15.1 Different types of exercise that might be recommended for you following assessment by a physiotherapist

* **General exercises,** for your overall fitness.
* **Cardiovascular exercises** to improve your heart rate, blood pressure and circulation.
* **Stretching exercises** to reduce the risk of spasticity and contractures – these work by stretching muscles and tendons to increase their flexibility and elasticity.
* **Resistance exercises**, using weights or other devices, to help increase muscle strength.
* **Motion exercises** to improve joint movements, reduce joint stiffness and tendon and ligament problems.

My wife has MS. Are there any special things I should do or avoid doing when I help her with the exercises recommended by the physiotherapist?

As far as possible your wife should aim to do the exercises every day, or as frequently as the physiotherapist has recommended. She can always opt out if she is having a particularly bad day or is feeling unwell. She should try to do the exercises at a time of day when she is not too tired, and when she has time to rest afterwards – she

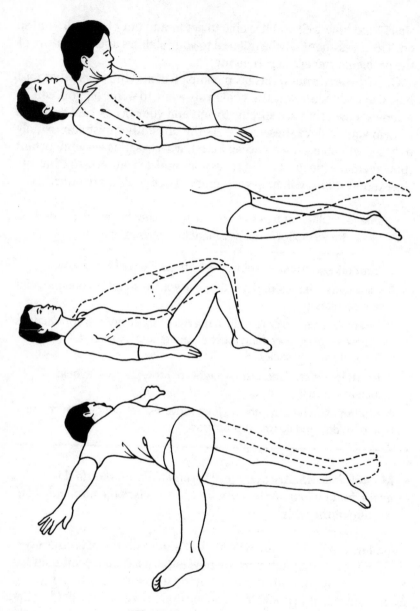

Figure 15.1 Floor exercises

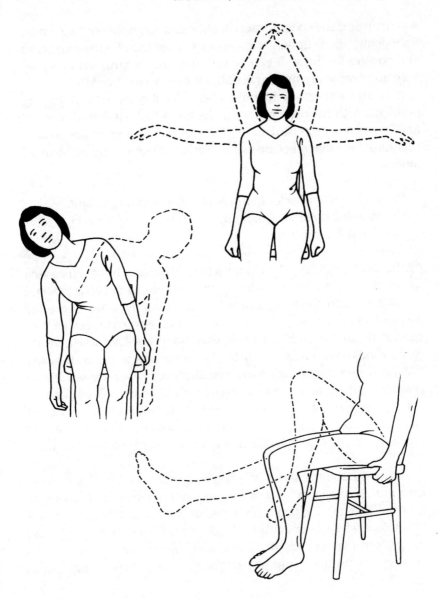

Figure 15.2 Chair exercises

will struggle if she does the exercises immediately before setting out on a shopping trip. Your wife is also likely to need lots of encouragement and positive feedback. It can be very difficult for anyone to keep up with an exercise regime, particularly if that person has MS.

It is also important to remember that if your wife is having problems with the exercises, or if she has a bad patch with her MS and has to stop exercising for a time, she should contact her physiotherapist for advice because the exercise regime may need to be modified.

Quite often the muscles in my legs stiffen up and go rigid. I believe this is called spasticity. I can't move and it's very painful. What can I do?

The term *spasticity* refers to muscle stiffness that has been caused by damage to nerve pathways in the central nervous system. Spasticity affects the legs more commonly than the arms. It is quite common in MS and it may cause spasms that, as you say, can be very painful. Regular stretching exercises are often beneficial and there are medications which may also help. It is important to know there are certain things which can make spasticity worse – poor seating or posture, clothing or shoes which are too tight or are rubbing, constipation, bladder infection, ingrowing toenails and pressure sores. If you think any of these factors may be causing problems, it will certainly help if you can tackle them. Ask for help from your MS nurse or GP.

One of the complications which can sometimes occur if you suffer from increased tone in some of your muscles is that contractures may develop. This can happen if the muscles become shortened and can lead to considerable discomfort if not tackled. The best way to avoid contractures is to make sure you maintain stretching exercises and keep a good posture – your physiotherapist can help with this.

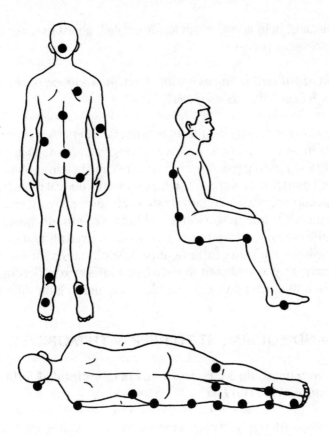

Figure 15.3 Areas where pressure sores can develop

I keep being told that posture is important. Why is this?

Anyone with poor posture may find they are more vulnerable to aches and pains, move more awkwardly and have difficulty breathing deeply and eating properly. All of these things also apply to someone with MS. If you have poor posture, you are more likely to be putting strain on different joints in the body and this can cause pain. If this is not sorted out, it may lead to osteoarthritis. Your physiotherapist can help and give advice, if needed, about managing and improving your posture.

What about swimming as a way of getting some exercise even though I can't do this very well?

Swimming is an excellent form of exercise. It enables your whole body to get a workout as well as ensuring you are supported in the water, thereby easing pressure on your joints and helping you to relax. It doesn't matter that you can't swim very well. You will probably find that you can only swim a relatively short distance anyway. Just being able to move around in the water will help. Swimming can be quite tiring and so can getting out of the pool, showering and dressing afterwards. If you think this might be difficult, make sure you take someone with you and plan to have a rest afterwards. Getting a lift home for a sit down and a hot chocolate can make all the difference!

AIDS AND EQUIPMENT TO HELP WITH MOBILITY

I am very unsteady on my legs, and I'm now afraid of falling in my house. What can I do?

It sounds as though you need a reassessment of your condition and your circumstances – there are several different people who can help and you should contact either your MS nurse or GP to get things moving. If you have an MS nurse, he or she can assess whether there are any interventions that may help your balance and walking ability – particularly if this is a recent change. You may need to be referred to the local rehabilitation team, which consists of several different professionals. The most relevant of these to your current circumstances will be the physiotherapist and occupational therapist.

The physiotherapist will assess you to see if there are any exercises, walking aids or other therapies which may help you get around more safely. The physiotherapist may visit together with the occupational therapist, who will be looking at the problems you have around the house and can arrange for various aids and adaptations which you may find useful. An extra stair rail, a grab rail next to the toilet, or a perching stool to use in the kitchen may all be helpful.

The physiotherapist and occupational therapist can also work with you to help find the best and safest way to get up again in case you fall. This can often relieve any anxiety you may have and help you feel more in control again. A pendant alarm which you can wear round your neck may be recommended. This connects you to a designated person when activated so that if you do fall you can easily get someone to come and help.

Housework is becoming a big problem because I have had to change so much to make it safe for me and I can't actually do it all. What should I do?

Housework is often a problem, not just in the practical sense of whether or not people can still do it, but also because it can cause a lot of anxiety and stress, particularly to women. If you have always been the one who has done the bulk of the housework, and who gets the most satisfaction from having a clean and tidy house, it can be hugely frustrating when this becomes more difficult to achieve.

From a practical point of view it is important to get some help. You may be able to apportion jobs between family members, making sure everyone is clear what you are asking them to do and when. Friends and other family members may also be willing to come and help out from time to time. Some people take the option of paying for a cleaner to come in once or twice a week and this can be very helpful, especially if you don't have many friends or family members around who are able to contribute. It is also important, but often really hard, to 'let go' a little. It is usually the case that, despite their best efforts, other people are unable to clean your house to the standard you would like. But the important thing to remember is that it *is* getting cleaned. If your energy is limited, there may be far more worthwhile things to spend it on than washing up.

Other people who may be able to help you manage the housework more easily are occupational therapists. They can provide all sorts of aids and adaptations which can make your life much easier. So talk to family and friends and also contact your MS nurse or occupational therapist to see what help and suggestions they can offer to make your housework less of a struggle.

I'm having increasing problems getting in and out of my bath and on and off the toilet. I find asking my husband to help rather undignified. What else can I do?

These sorts of problems can usually be solved relatively easily. The best person to help is your occupational therapist who can visit you at home, identify the particular difficulties you are having, and advise you about the various aids and adaptations which can help you to be more independent. These may include a grab rail next to the toilet and modified seating in the bathroom (some examples of these are shown in Figure 15.4). Once you have agreed the equipment that will be most useful, they will arrange for it to be delivered and fitted – there may be a small charge for this service.

I have a lot of trouble with dressing. Do you have any tips for me?

This can be a very frustrating problem, especially when you are in a hurry, but there are quite a few things that can be done to help. One of the simplest is to change the type of clothes you wear – at least on the days you don't have too much planned. Try to make sure you avoid anything with fiddly buttons or tight waistbands: tops that can go on straight over your head and pull-on skirts or trousers are often easiest. Your occupational therapist may be able to help with these sorts of problems, and even provide equipment that makes dressing much easier – such as gadgets to get shoes and socks or tights on, and to fasten bras. Occupational therapists can also give more general advice about techniques you can use to make dressing easier.

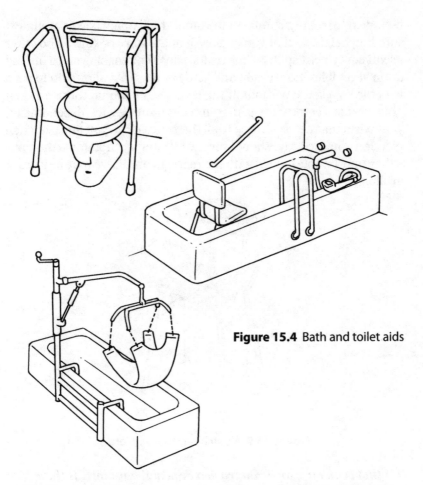

Figure 15.4 Bath and toilet aids

Working in the kitchen is now proving very difficult. Is it worth having the kitchen redesigned, or is there a less drastic solution?

Although a kitchen redesign may be the best solution in some circumstances, many people will find there are plenty of less drastic measures they can try first. You can start by talking to your occupational therapist, who will know about all sorts of equipment that can help you manage more easily in the kitchen. This may include a 'perching stool' – a tall stool that supports you at almost standing height so that you can use it at the stove or sink – and other useful equipment such as inserts for pans that enable you to lift and drain vegetables more easily, and kettle tippers that allow you to pour water from a kettle without lifting it up. Occupational therapists can also provide electric can openers and lots more besides, depending on your particular needs. If, despite all these measures, you find a kitchen redesign is needed, you should still involve your occupational therapist – they may be able to help with the redesign and there may be a grant available.

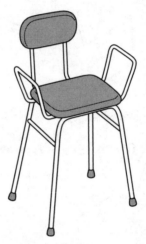

Figure 15.5 A perching stool with arms

I find I can't use an ordinary pen or pencil anymore. Is there anything else that would help me?

There are lots of different products on the market – many of which are available on the high street. Look for a pen with a large grip – it may be a matter of trying a few before you find one that suits you. Another option is to look for grips which can be slipped onto pens and pencils which you already have. The Disabled Living Foundation or Independent Living stores should have a selection you can choose from. If you can't find anything suitable, contact your MS nurse or occupational therapist and ask for help.

CHAIRS AND WHEELCHAIRS

The last thing I want to do is to use a wheelchair, but I think I am going to have to consider it. Do I really have to?

This is usually a difficult decision to make and one which many people put off for as long as possible. Always remember that a wheelchair is just a tool and a means to an end – it allows you to go to places you couldn't get to otherwise, and to be in a fit state to enjoy where you are going when you get there. What is the point of arriving at a lovely destination and being so shattered that you want to go straight home again?

Many people with MS own a wheelchair which they keep under the stairs or in the boot of the car for occasional use only – to be used when they are having a bad day, or if they want to go somewhere that they will struggle to get to otherwise. If you are at the stage where you are beginning to think about getting a wheelchair, it is probably a good time to get one. You can use it just when you need to and this will give you time to adjust to the idea. In this way, you can learn to use a wheelchair as it is meant to be used – to help you stay in control of where and when you go out, and to manage your fatigue and other symptoms more effectively.

When do you think that I should get a wheelchair?

You should get a wheelchair when you find that you are restricted in terms of where you can go or how long you can stay once you get there. Getting into a wheelchair for the first time is often very difficult psychologically, and people usually try to avoid doing this for as long as possible. One way to get over this first hurdle is to choose somewhere you really want to go that isn't local and where you are unlikely to bump into people you may know – go with your partner or a good friend, and use your wheelchair to enjoy the day out in order to make the whole experience positive and one you will want to repeat.

DRIVING

What help is available for drivers?

The help available depends on the specific problems you are having. As this is very individual, your MS nurse and occupational therapist are probably the best people to ask initially. The Motability Scheme is available to help people who are receiving the highest rate of the mobility component of Disability Living Allowance. The scheme enables disabled people to have a car adapted to their needs and is available to drivers and passengers alike. For example, hand controls can be made to operate foot pedals and certain types of vehicle can be adapted to allow you to get into your car without having to get out of your wheelchair. There are also driving assessment centres around the country that allow you to try different types of controls, and these centres can also give advice about the sort of adaptations that may be helpful.

My wife has difficulty getting in and out of our car. I don't want to buy another one at present. What can I do to help her?

The first thing to do is to ask for help as there may be a number of reasons why this is becoming more of a problem. Your MS nurse, physiotherapist and occupational therapist can all help with this and may be able to solve the problem by showing your wife different ways of getting in and out of the car, by treating the cause of her difficulties (for example, spasticity and spasms), or by providing equipment such as a swivel cushion or a handle which can be attached to the outside of the car when required to enable her to get in and out. If your wife's problems are more complex, there are a whole range of other car

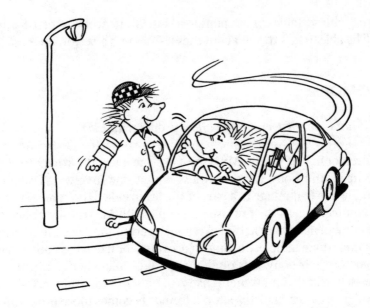

adaptations which may be helpful. Your occupational therapist will be able to advise you about these but they may be costly.

I am worried that my driving licence might be taken away because I have MS. Should I be concerned?

When you are diagnosed with MS, it is important that you notify both the Driver and Vehicle Licensing Agency (DVLA) and your insurance company, as you are bound to do so by law. As long as you are still safe to drive – which is the case for the vast majority of people with MS – you should not have any restrictions applied to your standard driving licence (Group 1 entitlement). However, if you hold a PSV or HGV licence (Group 2 entitlement) the regulations are much stricter and you will need to check with the DVLA directly.

You may need to stop driving if your vision is affected or if you are unable to use the hand controls or foot pedals properly. Coming to terms with this decision is always hard, although a matter of common-sense given the risks involved. It may be possible for you to start driving again with suitable car adaptations. Your GP, neurologist or MS nurse will be able to talk to you about these issues and give you their advice.

TREMOR

What types of tremor can affect people with MS?

Tremor in people with MS is most likely to affect the arms – the legs, head and body are much less commonly involved. Tremor is usually due to damage to a part of the brain called the cerebellum, or its connections in the brainstem. People with MS usually notice the tremor when they are actively keeping a part of their body in a certain position – for example, holding an arm out – or when they are moving a part of their body. It is often most noticeable when performing a precisely directed movement, like reaching out for an object. As the hand gets closer to its target, the tremor becomes more pronounced (this is called an intention tremor). This sort of tremor is quite different from the type that occurs in Parkinson's disease, which is most evident at rest and usually disappears with movement.

Are there any proven treatments for tremor?

A very disabling tremor is not often seen in people with MS. This is just as well because treatment is difficult and usually quite disappointing. It is rare for drugs to be beneficial. Propanolol can sometimes help a little, and other drugs including gabapentin, clonazepam, ondansetron, topiramate, isoniazid and primidone have all been reported to improve tremor occasionally. Neurologists are generally very cautious and unenthusiastic about prescribing these medications because so few people seem to benefit and because of the risk of troublesome side effects. Although splinting an affected limb, or attaching small weights to clothes to damp down tremor is sometimes tried, these measures are usually of only limited benefit, particularly if the limb is weak as well as tremulous.

When a person is very severely affected by tremor, there may sometimes be a role for carefully guided brain surgery. Some studies have shown that making a tiny scar (thalamotomy), or placing a stimulating electrode (thalamic stimulation), in a part of the brain called the thalamus may sometimes help. There will only be a handful of people with MS for whom this sort of procedure will be appropriate and the benefits may only be temporary. It is very important this sort of brain surgery is only performed by neurosurgeons who are experienced in these procedures, in order to improve the chance of a good outcome and reduce the risk of complications, including visual and speech problems.

16 | Speech problems, swallowing difficulties, and diet

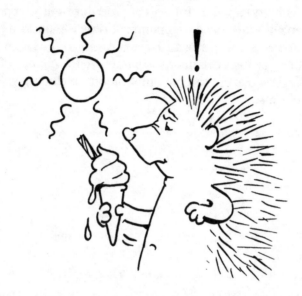

Problems with speech or with swallowing are fairly common among people living with MS, though not necessarily both together. In this chapter we address both these problems and discuss the different things that can be done to help. We also look at some of the different supplements and the different dietary advice available and try to make some sensible suggestions as to what you can best do to help keep yourself as well as possible.

SPEECH

While difficulty with speech is perhaps one of the more obvious problems you might face at some point, speech is only one of the ways in which we communicate. Facial expression, body movement and posture are all linked with speech, in order to communicate our thoughts and needs. Nevertheless, speech itself can often be the focus of concern, both for people with MS and their loved ones.

MS has the potential to affect the control of most muscles, so it is not surprising that it can affect those muscles that control voice production. As with other symptoms of MS, problems with speech can vary, particularly in the earlier stages of the disease. Although speech difficulties cannot currently be remedied by curing the under-lying neurological problem, appropriate advice, support and exercises can improve things considerably.

People say to me, 'Are you drunk?' I know that's what I sound like when my voice is bad, but how can I overcome this?

Slurred speech or speech that is difficult to understand is fairly common in MS and tends to be worse when you are feeling tired, or are stressed, anxious or feeling otherwise unwell. It can be hard to cope with – especially when others don't understand and jump to wild conclusions. There are, however, things you can do that might help. Talk to your MS nurse or neurologist who can refer you to a speech therapist. This is likely to be very helpful.

A speech therapist will assess the extent of the problem and then give you a series of exercises and advice specific to your particular problems. This will help and should restore some of your confidence which may well have been damaged in a 'vicious circle'. You may feel stressed and worked up when your speech is slurred, and the stress itself can then make your speech even worse, which then makes you feel even more frustrated – and so on. A speech therapist can help you to break this cycle, and give you advice about how to speak more slowly and calmly so that what you say is easier for others to understand.

EATING AND SWALLOWING

Will I develop problems eating or swallowing?

Between 30 and 40 per cent of people with MS are likely to develop problems with eating and swallowing. The majority of people with these symptoms will just experience difficulty with coughing or spluttering when eating or drinking. Drinking often causes more problems than eating as thicker, textured foods and drinks (see below) are easier to swallow.

Like many other symptoms of MS, problems with swallowing can come and go and will be worse when you are tired or unwell or worked up about something. If you think you are developing problems, then do talk to your neurologist or MS nurse. You may be referred to a speech and language therapist for advice as these professionals deal with swallowing problems as well as with difficulties with speech.

I have real problems swallowing solid food. What can I do about it?

The first thing to do is to ask for help. Contact one of the health professionals with whom you are in touch and tell them about the problems you are having. This will enable you to be referred to a speech and language therapist who is trained to help deal with swallowing problems as well as problems specifically related to speech.

In the meantime, there are plenty of things you can do yourself that will help. Like most symptoms of MS, swallowing problems are at their worst when you are tired, unwell or feeling emotional; try to identify triggers that make the problem worse for you. Examples might include types of food or liquid, or particular drink containers. If you identify that swallowing is more difficult at particular times of the day, try to avoid eating much at these times or change the type of food you are eating. For example, some people change the time of their main meal from evening to lunchtime when they are less tired, then just have a light meal in the evening. Others find they prefer their main meal in the evening as they feel better after a rest in the afternoon. Think about what works best for you and your family.

Try to ensure you are sitting in as upright a position as possible when you are eating. Try to keep your chin tucked in as this ensures your oesophagus is nicely aligned. When swallowing, make sure that you have cleared each mouthful of food or drink from your mouth and throat before taking another.

The type of food you are eating may also make a difference – softer textured foods may well be a good choice when you are having a bad day or are very tired. If drinks are causing you difficulty (and often they can be more of a problem than more solid foods) try drinks with added texture such as smoothies, pulped orange juice or milk shakes.

When you see a speech therapist, he or she will be able to make a proper assessment of your swallowing problems and give you expert advice specific to your circumstances.

Why do I have the same problem swallowing liquids?

As mentioned in the previous answer, liquids can actually be more difficult to swallow than solids. There may be particular difficulty with liquids that are less thick and 'dense'. This is because the liquids pass through the mouth 'too fast' before the slower moving muscles have a chance to coordinate swallowing, so there is a risk of coughing and choking, as liquids might run into the airway to the lungs. Usually this problem is solved by thickening the liquids, so that they pass through the mouth more slowly and stand a far greater chance of being swallowed. Try some if these suggestions, and those mentioned in the previous answer. Do discuss any continuing problems with your MS nurse.

Why does MS cause some people to vomit?

It is unusual for people with MS to vomit, although a feeling of nausea (wanting to vomit without ever quite getting there) is more common. Both symptoms tend to be associated with vertigo which is a feeling of dizziness or of your surroundings moving without you.

If you are experiencing these symptoms have a chat with your GP, neurologist or MS nurse as they will be able to suggest a variety of different medications which may help.

DIET AND MS

How do your views on diet differ from those of the MS Society? Does diet have an impact on MS?

Our views don't really differ from the MS Society and we often use their leaflets about diet when giving information to the people with MS that we see.

We advise people to follow a normal healthily balanced diet – try to make sure you get your five portions of fruit and vegetables each day, and choose food from across the different food groups of meat or fish, fatty/sugary foods, fruit and vegetables, dairy and carbohydrates. If you can manage to balance your dietary intake across these groups, enjoying as much variety as you can, you should find that you are eating well and getting all the vitamins and nutrients you need. People who follow vegetarian or vegan diets should aim to do the same using vegetable protein to replace the meat and fish.

Some experts feel it may be helpful if you can cut down the amount of meat that you eat and increase the amount of oily fish (for example, salmon, mackerel, sardines and tuna). This is because it is thought to be helpful to reduce animal (or saturated) fat, even though there is no robust research to support this notion. At the very least, it is well known that unsaturated fats are less harmful than saturated, particularly to the heart and blood circulation.

Is Vitamin B12 linked to MS?

MS is a condition that causes loss of myelin insulation (demyelination) around the nerve cells. Vitamin B12 is needed by your body to make myelin and very low levels can cause symptoms similar to those experienced in MS. These observations have led, understandably, to suggestions that vitamin B12 may be a useful treatment for MS. However, research does not support this theory; the vast majority of people with MS have a normal vitamin B12 level and if a deficiency is detected, it is most likely to be a coincidental finding. You do not need to have your vitamin B12 level checked just because you have MS. However, it is appropriate to do this test if you are anaemic, have a poor diet or are unable to absorb food properly. If you have any concerns, your doctor can check your vitamin B12 levels. If the test result is satisfactory, you will not need treatment. Although some people with MS do have regular vitamin B12 injections and claim that they feel better as a result, there is little evidence to support this approach. Remember that a proportion of people will feel better on placebo (dummy drug). We therefore do not recommend vitamin B12 injections in people with MS who have normal vitamin B12 levels.

I've heard foods rich in vitamin B are good for you. Which sources of food should I eat to maintain a healthy central nervous system?

Cheese, milk, nuts and grains are all good sources of vitamin B, as are green vegetables. The B vitamins are thought to be important for nerve cell health. Vitamin B12, in particular, is known to be necessary in the formation of the myelin that surrounds nerve cells. However, there is no convincing evidence that treatment with B vitamins is helpful for MS, in itself.

I've heard low vitamin D levels can cause MS. Is this true?

Vitamin D is needed to keep your bones strong and prevent them from becoming thin and brittle. One of the main sources is from exposure of your skin to the sun. It has been suggested that vitamin D deficiency may be linked with MS. This theory is supported by the fact that MS is more common the further you get from the equator where there is less sunlight. Although this is an attractive hypothesis, there are other possible environmental and genetic explanations for the geographical distribution of MS across the globe. Also, vitamin D dietary supplements have not been shown to be beneficial and routine treatment cannot be recommended for MS. However, you might need treatment with vitamin D, calcium and other medications if you have significant bone thinning (osteoporosis) due to your age or excessive treatment with steroids.

What about vitamin and mineral supplements? I am sure that I have read that people with MS have deficiencies in some key vitamins and minerals. Wouldn't it be good to take those?

If you are eating a varied and well-balanced diet you shouldn't need to take any supplements as you will get all the vitamins and minerals you need through your diet. The only dietary supplement recommended by NICE (the National Institute for Health and Clinical Excellence) is 17–23 g linoleic acid, although this is not based on cast iron evidence as none exists. Sources of linoleic acid include sunflower or safflower oil, and nuts (including walnuts, brazil nuts, pine nuts and almonds). Some people choose to take vitamin supplements on a daily basis, even though this isn't strictly necessary, because they feel this will ensure they are getting the recommended daily amount they need.

If you have to follow a restricted diet for some reason, then you should take the advice of your dietitian or MS nurse.

If you have problems with poor digestion, is it linked to poor mobility or something you have from the start?

Problems with poor digestion are common and are not always related to MS – many people who don't have MS experience difficulties. Food is moved from the stomach, through the intestines, by a process known as peristalsis where muscles in the wall of the gut contract, squeezing the food along rather like toothpaste in a tube. Just as muscles in your legs can become weak or prone to spasm, so can the muscles in the gut. This can make the time taken for food to travel through the gut much longer than is comfortable and lead to you feeling bloated and generally uncomfortable.

Poor mobility can exacerbate existing problems with poor digestion and reviewing your dietary and fluid intake can help, as can taking other forms of exercise that don't involve you standing up. Your GP or local nurse can give you lots of advice about this.

If I decide to have additional essential fatty acids in my diet, what should I take?

We do not yet know for certain whether essential fatty acids help MS although they may have anti-inflammatory and immuno-suppressant properties. Essential fatty acids serve as a source of energy as well as helping to store certain vitamins. NICE recommends that people with MS should take between 17–23 g of linoleic acid 'to help reduce the disabling effects of MS'. However, the evidence that linoleic acid can have a significant impact on MS is not robust. It appears that Omega-6 and Omega-3 may be important essential fatty acids and, if you follow a healthy balanced diet, then you should take in plenty of these naturally without the need for dietary supplements.

I have heard about something called an 'exclusion diet' for MS. Is it likely to help?

The short answer is no! Any diet which excludes significant food groups can only result in an unbalanced diet which will be lacking in essential nutrients. There is no evidence that exclusion diets help with MS and they can result in people suffering deficiencies of key nutrients.

In the past certain exclusion diets have gained a reputation for helping with MS and it is understandable how this can happen. MS is so variable and each individual's symptoms differ, often on a daily basis. This inevitably means that, if a good period coincides with starting a new dietary regime or excluding a certain food group, it is very tempting to attribute the improvement to the changes. In truth it is likely that the improvement would have occurred anyway and the link with a change in diet is purely coincidental. This is why it is always important to subject any new treatments or theories to rigorous scientific study, in order to exclude any effects of coincidence or random variability.

If you feel that MS will not necessarily be affected by dietary change, what would you suggest I do in relation to eating and drinking?

As discussed above, a healthy balanced diet is important for all of us in ensuring our general health and the more you can do to look after yourself generally, the less likely you are to develop other problems in addition to MS – which is the last thing anyone wants. So it is still well worth following a healthy eating plan and enjoying a varied, balanced diet. The occasional treat is allowed too though!

Does MS make you get drunk quicker?

It does in a way. Many people with MS find that they are more sensitive to alcohol and that they can only tolerate a couple of drinks when perhaps they used to be able to drink more than this without feeling the effects. Alcohol tends to exaggerate the symptoms of clumsiness and unsteadiness that many people with MS already have. If you alternate alcoholic drinks with non-alcoholic ones, or just make sure you drink plenty of water at the same time, then you should still be able to enjoy a night out without too many ill effects.

Is it usual to lose weight without trying to do so?

Some people do lose weight, particularly if they have more severe MS and have difficulty eating or a marked tremor. However, some people with MS experience weight loss that can't be easily explained. If this happens to you, it is important that you have a chat with your GP, neurologist or MS nurse. They will want to look at what you are eating and drinking each day and to get some idea of the amount of weight you have lost over a given time period. They may also look at the medications you are taking to make sure your weight loss is not a side effect of your tablets. In addition, they will want to know about your bowel habits to get some idea of how efficiently you are absorbing your food. If you are still losing weight at a significant rate and there is no obvious cause, your GP or neurologist may want to do some more investigations to rule out problems unconnected with MS. They may be happy to refer you to a dietitian for advice and monitoring of the weight loss, or they may wish to monitor the situation over time.

While you should always get professional advice about unexplained weight loss, there are some things you can do to help yourself. Sometimes fatigue can mean that you are so tired by the time you come to eat that you just don't fancy the food anymore – particularly if you have had to prepare the meal yourself. Try eating your main meal at lunchtime when you are less tired. Make sure your kitchen is adapted to make life as easy as possible for you – contact your occupational therapist if this is a problem. You may be able to make meals with two to three extra servings at a time, and freeze these extra portions so you can just reheat them if you are feeling tired rather than having to prepare anything from scratch. It is even better if you can get someone else to prepare some meal portions for you and stock up the freezer! If eating a big meal is too off-putting, eating little and often throughout the day can ensure you get the calories, energy and nutrients you need – try to plan your eating for the day to make sure you get a good balance of the different food groups. Dietary supplements can provide extra calories as well as other nutrients and are always worth considering – your dietitian or MS nurse can advise you on their use.

17 | Problems with eyesight and hearing

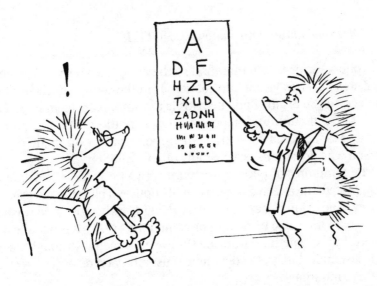

Visual problems are common in MS and for some may be one of the first presenting signs of MS. More rarely, some people with MS experience problems with their hearing. This chapter explores some of the problems you might encounter and discusses what can be done to help.

EYE PROBLEMS

My eyesight is getting worse, and is very bad when my MS is bad. Why is this?

Typically, visual problems come and go – although a proportion of people are left with permanent damage of varying degrees. If your vision is affected by your MS, it is likely to be particularly sensitive to your general health and mood and many people comment that their vision deteriorates when they are tired, stressed or unwell. You should discuss this with your MS nurse or neurologist if it is a recurring problem.

I have read about optic neuritis. What is it?

Optic neuritis is inflammation in the optic (eye) nerve. The optic nerve carries visual information from the retina, at the back of the eye, to the brain. Optic neuritis is a common problem in people with MS, but can also happen in other conditions that sometimes mimic MS. Sometimes, optic neuritis can happen on its own in a person who doesn't have MS or any other condition.

The symptoms of optic neuritis are fairly characteristic. As might be expected, the affected person usually notices a blurring of vision in one eye and colours may be less vivid, looking rather grey and washed out. There may also be pain in or behind the eye. This is usually not severe, but is sometimes worsened by eye movement. Although vision is occasionally badly affected, there is usually good recovery over two to three months.

What is happening when I have double vision, or when my vision is wobbly?

Double vision happens when both eyes are not moving in unison, so that images are not properly aligned. In people with MS, this happens because of damage to the nerve connections (neural pathways) involved in the control of the eye muscles. If double vision has come on recently – as in the case of a brainstem relapse – an eye patch may be used as a short-term measure pending recovery. If double vision has been a problem for many weeks or months, and is not changing, referral to an eye specialist may be needed. Special prismatic glasses that correct the alignment of the images may be helpful.

Wobbly vision, or oscillopsia, occurs when disturbance of the control of eye movements results in the eyes bobbing up and down or from side to side. These abnormal eye movements are called nystagmus and typically happen – as does double vision – when the brainstem is involved. If this occurs as a consequence of recent inflammation (a brainstem relapse), spontaneous recovery may occur and this process may be speeded by treatment with steroids. If the problem is long-standing, treatment may be very difficult although some medications may occasionally be of benefit.

Can glasses help double vision and eyestrain?

Double vision and eyestrain are not necessarily the same thing. Eye tiredness may well be helped by glasses, though it depends on what is causing it. Everyone should have regular check-ups with an optician anyway, regardless of whether or not they have MS. This will detect any changes in your eyes that can be helped by glasses and may well solve any problems of eyestrain.

Double vision is usually a temporary problem that comes and goes. Many people find that wearing a patch over one eye can make things a bit easier to manage when doing close work, using a computer or watching television. If the problem has developed recently, it may be a symptom of relapse and treatment with steroids may speed recovery. If the double vision is not resolving, referral to a specialist eye doctor (ophthalmologist) may be helpful. Although double vision will not usually be helped by wearing standard prescription glasses, prism spectacles may be beneficial.

PROBLEMS WITH HEARING

Does MS affect your hearing?

Hearing loss is not one of the common problems associated with MS but a few people do develop symptoms of hearing impairment and very rarely can develop quite profound difficulties. Given that hearing loss is unusual in MS, it is always worth discussing the problem with your GP. It may be due to something very simple such as a build up of wax or some other cause unrelated to MS. Your GP or neurologist may refer you to an ear specialist if the cause of your problems is uncertain.

18 | Sexual function

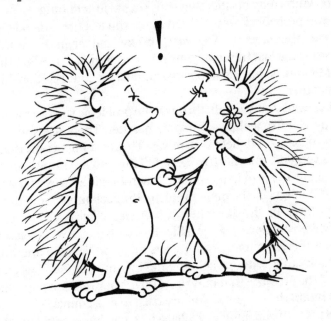

Sexual difficulties can be a part of anyone's life and are not helped by MS – which can certainly complicate things! In this chapter we try to address problems which may be caused directly by MS such as lack of sensation or erectile dysfunction; we also look at problems caused indirectly by MS such as the impact of fatigue or spasticity on sexual function, and finally we have tried to look more broadly to touch on the impact of sexual difficulties on relationships and the help that is available.

Can MS affect your sexual libido? And, if so, can you get anything on prescription for it?

MS can certainly affect your libido and it can do so for a number of reasons. However, it is also important to remember that not every problem you experience with your sex drive will be a direct consequence of MS. It is always important to rule out any other factors which may be affecting your sexual functioning.

As you probably know, MS can make you feel tired, moody and fed up. It can also make you feel very 'unsexy' and mean that wanting to have sex is the last thing on your mind! Indeed, just the fact that you have MS may be having a negative impact on your relationship with your partner.

It is crucial that you talk through the problems you are having and the way you are feeling with your partner. There are some simple things you can do to help yourselves. The most important thing is to ensure you and your partner keep talking and are honest with each other about the problems you are having and the way you are both feeling. If fatigue is the main problem, think about making time to be close at times of the day when you are less likely to be tired. Many couples who are having some difficulties with their sexual relationship find that there are many other ways they can be close and intimate with each other without actually having intercourse. This can ease some of the pressure that may build up in your relationship, allowing you to retain the closeness you are used to as a couple.

There is no medication available which can improve libido for either men or women; there are treatments available if you are unable to get or to maintain an erection and these are discussed later in this chapter. Other types of help include treatment of MS-specific symptoms (such as fatigue, spasm, lack of bladder control) which may be hindering your sex drive, or specialist counselling (including couples' counselling) to help you deal with any concerns such as low self-esteem, poor body image and relationship problems which are relatively common in MS.

It may be worth seeking advice from a healthcare professional you both feel able to talk to about this sensitive issue – your MS nurse or GP are often the first port of call. They can help you put things in perspective and may be able to help with some of the difficulties you are experiencing and arrange referral for specialist help if needed.

As a relatively young man with MS, I am sure that I am having some sexual problems that I reckon are due to the MS. Do you think that's likely?

Depending upon which study you read, up to 50 per cent of people (1 in 2) with MS will have sexual problems at some stage in their condition. Some may be the direct result of MS, such as difficulty achieving and/or maintaining an erection. Others may have a more indirect cause due to fatigue, spasticity, bladder problems and low mood. MS can also change the way people feel about themselves and their partner, and this can have an adverse affect on a sexual relationship. It is also important to be aware that not all sexual problems are linked to MS. Approximately 40 per cent (2 in 5) of the general population will have sexual problems at some time in their life.

I'm really having difficulty 'performing' sexually and most of the time I can't get an erection. What is the problem?

Difficulty achieving and maintaining an erection is known as erectile dysfunction. This is very common in MS and can be caused directly by damage to the nerve connections between the brain, spinal cord and penis. It can also be due to indirect causes including fatigue, low mood and bladder problems. MS can also contribute to relationship problems that may adversely affect sexual functioning. There are a number of other possible causes unrelated to MS, including blood circulation problems, so it is important that you talk to your GP.

A great deal of help is available to improve sexual performance, so do talk to your GP or MS nurse about the difficulties you are having. The following answers may also be of interest as they give information about the different medications which can be used to treat erectile dysfunction as well as some of the other types of help available.

I really don't feel like having sex any more. Is this the result of my MS? I am worried that my relationship with my husband is now deteriorating badly as a result. What can I do?

This is a very common problem and lots of people – men as well as women – feel like this at some stage. Many people without MS also experience periods like this in their sexual relationships, although having MS certainly doesn't help. MS can make you feel very tired, moody and depressed. It can also affect the way you feel about yourself and erode your self confidence and self-esteem so that the last thing you feel is sexy. MS might be affecting the way you feel about your husband – if he now has to give you more help with things like getting dressed, going to the toilet, or is just having to take on more responsibility for the day-to-day running of the household, you might be feeling as though your role within the home and within your relationship has changed for the worse. Talk to your husband about how you are feeling and consider seeking some professional help.

There are a number of different approaches which can be helpful in resolving problems with sexual functioning depending on your individual concerns and problems. Some people find that problems caused directly by MS (for example symptoms such as poor bladder control, spasm, tremor and fatigue) are affecting their sexual relationship. Treatment for these may help to ease the problems they are causing in your sexual relationship.

MS can also result in loss of sensation in different parts of the body, which can hinder arousal. There is a technique known as body mapping which can help couples to overcome these problems. This involves taking time together to find the areas of each others' bodies which respond to sensitive touch. There are specialist clinics available in most areas with specially trained doctors and counsellors who can help couples to overcome the problems they are facing using techniques such as body mapping. These clinics can be accessed via your GP, neurologist or MS nurse.

Some couples find specialist counselling can be very helpful in dealing with any emotional concerns they may have – for example, helping to overcome and work through feelings of low self-esteem, changes in role and loss of desire.

Both the MS Trust and the MS Society produce helpful booklets which give more information about tackling sexual difficulties in MS. See Appendix 1 for contact details.

I've heard a lot about Viagra for men's impotence. Could this help me sexually?

Sildenafil (Viagra) is just one of the medications now available to treat erectile dysfunction (the inability to get or maintain an erection). These medications can certainly help men to achieve an erection and are used with good effect by a significant number of people. However, the prescription of these medications is restricted and they are only available via your GP. The good news is that MS is one of the conditions for which GPs are allowed to prescribe them if they feel it may help.

The medications currently are available include sildenafil (Viagra), tadalafil (Cialis) and vardenafil (Levitra). These drugs all work in a similar way by ensuring that when the man is sexually aroused, blood vessels in the penis expand to produce an erection and remain expanded for longer to maintain the erection. However, these drugs have no effect if arousal doesn't occur.

These drugs should be used with caution. They can cause a drop in blood pressure (which makes some people feel dizzy) and if you are already taking medications to lower your blood pressure, drug treatment for erectile dysfunction may not be an option. Alcohol can also interact with these drugs and it does nothing to help improve your sexual performance. Grapefruit juice can also cause an increase in the effect of these medications and should not be taken at the same time. Common side effects include dizziness, headaches, indigestion and flushing. Occasionally, some men may find they experience prolonged and painful erections. If you experience an erection lasting four hours or more you should contact your local Accident and Emergency department for help and advice. Certain groups of people should not take these medications at all as they would be too much at risk from harmful effects. This includes anyone who has unstable angina or gets an angina attack during sex, anyone who has had a heart attack or stroke within the last six months, and anyone with uncontrolled blood pressure.

All this may sound quite daunting and off-putting, but many men do find these medications are helpful, and use them with few (if any) side effects. Don't forget to talk through the pros and cons of taking these tablets with your partner as well as your GP.

Can women benefit from Viagra as well as men?

There has been quite a lot of research done to find out whether medications such as sildenafil (Viagra) can help women to increase their likelihood of orgasm but unfortunately there appears to be no benefit. Sexual problems in women are much more difficult to treat than in men – perhaps because the female sexual response is more complex than that of men. Nevertheless, there are a number of things that can be tried and it is important to ask for help if you are struggling with this aspect of your relationship (see also the answer to two questions above). There is a good booklet produced by the MS Trust called 'Sexuality and MS: A Guide for Women', which is available free to order or download from the MS Trust website.

I have a problem with bladder incontinence. This is proving to be difficult for me to cope with, particularly when we want to have sex. Is there anything I can do?

This is quite a common problem and one shared by men and women. Fortunately, there is quite a lot you can do. The first and most important thing is to make sure you get some help and advice with managing your continence problems – these issues are addressed more fully in Chapter 12 on 'Bladder and bowels'.

In terms of what you can do to manage your bladder continence in relation to having sex, the following advice may be helpful. If you think that you and your husband may be going to make love, do everything you can to empty your bladder fully beforehand. It may also be worth reducing your fluid intake for a couple of hours beforehand but make sure to catch up with your daily intake later, otherwise you may become dehydrated. There are medications that can help provide you with better bladder control. Desmopressin is an anti-diuretic hormone that can be prescribed as a tablet or nasal spray, and can be taken overnight to reduce the amount of urine you produce. It is very important to talk to your husband about your problems, and the fears and anxieties you have about continence and lovemaking – hopefully, he will be able to reassure you. Just having a clean, soft towel around to place under you may be enough to ease any anxieties and alleviate your problems.

Recently, I have been finding lovemaking painful. What can I do?

There are lots of reasons why women can have pain during sexual intercourse – this is called dyspareunia. One of the most common reasons can be dryness of the vagina. Talk through the problems with your partner, encourage him to take his time and use lubricants. The onset of the menopause is also notorious for causing vaginal dryness, a problem which can often be easily remedied by the use of hormone replacement therapy (HRT). HRT can either be taken in tablet form or, if you prefer, used topically as a cream just to treat the vaginal dryness.

Other causes of dyspareunia include vaginismus (painful spasms of the vagina), problems with the cervix and infection. MS does not usually cause pain during sex although it can cause abnormal sensation down below. The treatment of nerve pain is addressed more fully in Chapter 13 on 'Pain, sensations, cramps and spasticity'. It is always worth seeking help and advice if you are experiencing pain during intercourse. Talk to your GP, or consult one of the other sources of help and advice such as a family planning clinic, a sexual health clinic, or your MS nurse.

The spasticity in my legs is a big problem when I try to have sexual intercourse. Is there any advice you can offer me about this?

This is quite a common problem and can be very off-putting (not to mention painful) for both you and your partner. However, spasticity and spasms can usually be managed fairly well. It may simply be a case of reducing aggravating factors, changing the dose of medication you are taking for spasticity, and experimenting to find the most comfortable position.

Your spasticity is likely to be more of a problem if you are very hot or tired, or have an infection, a full bladder or bowel, or are wearing tight clothing. It is therefore important to make sure you are comfortable, wear clothing which is light and not restrictive, or no clothing at all, and make sure you are able to keep cool – perhaps keep a window open or have a fan on. It also helps if you can make sure you go to the toilet beforehand.

If you are already taking medication to control spasticity, discuss the problems you are having with the person who prescribed your drug treatment. It may be helpful to adjust the dose or timing of the medication and sometimes taking an extra tablet before you have sex can solve the problem. If your spasticity and spasms remain a problem despite these measures, your MS nurse or GP should be able to advise whether referral to local rehabilitation services may be helpful.

Fatigue is my major problem when it comes to sex. I just don't feel I have the energy. What can I do?

Fatigue is a major problem for many people with MS and it can really interfere with your sex life! You may well have developed a routine of having sex at the same sort of time – typically people make love at the end of the day when they go to bed. It is very probable that this is the time of day when you are most tired and therefore least likely to feel like having sex. Talk to your partner and think about when you are least tired and most likely to have enough energy to enjoy having sex together. It may be that your fatigue levels are at their lowest in the morning and you can arrange to have some time alone together then. This might also mean that you can have a rest during the afternoon and then have enough energy to be able to enjoy the evening routine with your partner. There are also some other more general things you can do to tackle your fatigue and these are discussed in more detail in Chapter 14 on 'Fatigue, cognition and mood'.

I feel I am unusual as someone with MS who is gay. Almost all the advice I read about sexual relationships implies that people are heterosexual and are in opposite sex partnerships. Is there any recognition of the sexual problems gay people may have?

MS does not differentiate between people who are gay or straight and there are the same proportion of people who are gay, bisexual or transexual with MS as there are in the general population. Whatever your sexual orientation, the sexual advice that is available should still be relevant and will still apply to you. GLAMS (Gay men and Lesbians Affected by MS) is a self-help support group for gay and lesbian people with MS (see Appendix 1 for contact details). GLAMS provides information about living with MS and, more importantly, provides a forum for people to meet and share their experiences either at local meetings or on-line.

I am young and single. Most of the information available on sex seems to be for people who are in long-term relationships. Can you give me any advice?

Although most of the information is written as though it is aimed at people in long-term relationships, the actual advice will, for the most part, be relevant to you as well. The MS Trust produce a good booklet about sexual issues in MS and much of this is aimed just as much at young, single people as it is at well-established couples. As someone who is young and single, do enjoy it while it lasts! You should get on with your life and enjoy relationships in the same way as any other person of your age. If you are having difficulty with any aspects of sexual intercourse or your sexuality, then do ask for help from your GP or MS nurse – and try to talk to your partner about it.

19 | Pregnancy and childbirth

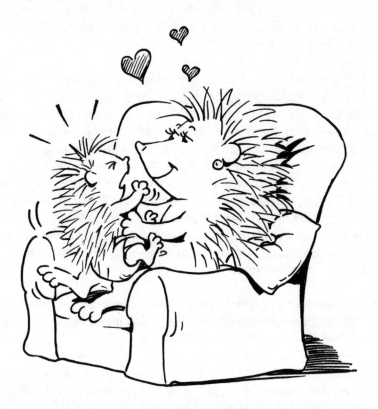

MS is often diagnosed when people are in their twenties or thirties and are either thinking about starting a family or may have recently had a child. Pregnancy and child birth is a common area of concern therefore for many people with MS, and perhaps also one of the areas where many misconceptions still abound.

In this chapter, we discuss all aspects of pregnancy from conception through to delivery and the impact of MS on this. We go on to explore the potential impact of MS after the birth of a child and what you can do to make this first year memorable for all the right reasons!

MS AND PREGNANCY

I have just been diagnosed with MS. What will the effect on my MS be if I have a baby?

Having a baby will not have any overall or long-term effect on your MS. Pregnancy itself leads to a dampening down of the immune system – this 'anti-inflammatory' state helps to stop the body rejecting the developing baby. As a result of this natural form of immuno-suppression, the chance of having a relapse actually goes down during pregnancy, particularly in the last three months (or third trimester). Unfortunately, this is followed by an increased risk in the first three months after delivery, which cancels out the benefit of the lower relapse rate during pregnancy. After this, the risk goes back to the pre-pregnancy level. As a consequence, there is no overall change in the number of relapses or any long-term effect on disability as a direct result of pregnancy.

My partner and I are hoping to start a family soon. What sort of issues would you advise me to think about before becoming pregnant, given that I have MS?

First of all, you should not forget the standard advice given to all women contemplating pregnancy. This includes taking folic acid to reduce the chance of neural tube defects (spina bifida), stopping smoking and reducing your alcohol intake. Secondly, it is important to consider the rate at which your MS has developed since you were diagnosed, and how you will be able to look after your children in the future. You should involve your partner, and perhaps your wider family, in these discussions. Thirdly, it is important to understand the effect pregnancy has on the risk of having a relapse and to discuss with your GP, neurologist or MS nurse what to do about any medication you may be taking. As a general rule, it is best to try to keep drug treatment to a minimum during pregnancy in order to reduce any risk to the baby. It is probably safe to use steroids for a relapse while you are pregnant, but best to avoid treatment in the first trimester if possible. It is also important to stop any disease-modifying drug before you try to get pregnant and restart it once you have given birth, providing you do not intend to breastfeed.

Although I have discussed the situation with my GP and neurologist, I am concerned about what my obstetrician might say about being pregnant with MS?

There is no medical reason to discourage you from considering a pregnancy simply because you have MS. Your obstetrician is very unlikely to advise you against getting pregnant. Your obstetrician or midwife may ask for advice from your neurologist or MS nurse but, in fact, no special precautions are needed. That said, it is sensible to agree a plan of action with your MS nurse in the unlikely event you have a relapse during pregnancy. It is probably safe to give steroids in the second and third trimester if you have a bad relapse, in order to speed recovery. You should be able to have a normal delivery unless there are other reasons why this may not be feasible.

Is it likely that a woman with MS will have any additional risks or problems in pregnancy or childbirth?

You are still at risk of having a relapse during pregnancy even though this risk is lower than before pregnancy – if you have a relapse it can be treated with steroids if needed. You may already feel fatigued and this may become more troublesome during pregnancy, but see Chapter 14 for more information on coping with this problem. Make sure you have adequate rest and try to improve the quality of your sleep. This may include treating bladder problems to avoid waking up to go the toilet in the night – reducing the amount of caffeine, alcohol and fluid you consume before going to bed may also help in this regard.

You should ensure that you do not skip meals – if there is no petrol in the car then the engine will not work! If you have a tendency towards anaemia, it would be sensible to discuss with your GP whether iron supplements are needed. Finally, you should be able to have a normal childbirth unless there are specific reasons, unrelated to your MS, why this may not be possible. You can have all the usual sorts of pain relief during delivery and there is no reason why you can't have an epidural for pain control if needed. If a caesarean is required, there is no extra risk to you because of the MS.

I am currently taking several drugs to combat the effects of the MS. Do I need to stop taking these if I decide to become pregnant?

The standard advice is to avoid any drug during pregnancy unless it is absolutely necessary. It is therefore a good idea to plan your pregnancy and discuss this specific issue with your GP, neurologist or MS nurse before you get pregnant. It is also important not to forget all the usual advice including taking folic acid to reduce the chance of neural tube defects (spina bifida), stopping smoking and moderating your alcohol consumption.

Always remember that reducing or stopping symptomatic drug treatment is not going to adversely affect the course of your MS, and that other non-drug treatments may be available for some of the symptoms you may be experiencing. Although steroids are not recommended in the first trimester, they can be used later in pregnancy if necessary. However, you may prefer to let any relapse improve spontaneously – avoiding steroids will not have a detrimental effect on the extent to which you recover from a relapse.

Disease-modifying drugs such as beta-interferon (Avonex, Betaferon, Extavia, Rebif 22/44), glatiramer acetate (Copaxone) and natalizumab (Tysabri) are not recommended for use in pregnancy and are probably best avoided. The number of pregnancies which have occurred in people receiving these treatments is small and so firm conclusions regarding their effects on the developing baby are difficult to establish. The available information indicates that there may be an increased risk of miscarriage in women on beta-interferon (Avonex,

Betaferon, Extavia, Rebif 22/44). One study suggested that exposure to beta-interferon during pregnancy was associated with low birth weight (similar to the effect of heavy smoking) and higher rates of miscarriage. Higher maternal age also increases the risk of losing a baby during pregnancy. It should be stressed, however, that the vast majority of women exposed to beta-interferon in early pregnancy give birth to normal healthy babies. There are over 1000 reports of pregnancies in women exposed to glatiramer acetate (Copaxone) and it does not appear to have any detrimental effects. Even so, the manufacturer recommends treatment should be stopped at least one full menstrual cycle before contraception is discontinued. It is important to restart the disease-modifying drug once you have given birth providing you do not intend to breastfeed, and remember to discuss contraception with your GP or family-planning nurse.

AFTER THE BIRTH

I have heard that relapses are more common after giving birth. Does this mean that I shouldn't have a baby?

No – although the risk of a relapse after giving birth increases for the first three months, it then returns to pre-pregnancy levels. The major predictive factor for having a relapse following childbirth is whether any relapses occurred in the year before pregnancy and during the pregnancy. That is, you are more likely to have a relapse following delivery if you have had a recent relapse, which is perhaps not surprising but certainly not a reason for not having a baby. If you were taking a disease-modifying drug before you got pregnant, it is important to restart treatment once you have delivered, providing you are not breastfeeding. That said, some women prefer to defer restarting treatment until they have stopped breastfeeding. It is also safe to have steroids if you have a bad relapse following childbirth.

Having an epidural does not increase the risk of having a relapse, and the length of time you've had MS, the sex of your baby, and the number of children you have already had does not have any influence either. Breastfeeding does not alter the risk of relapses and there is absolutely no risk of passing on MS to your baby through breast milk. The lifetime risk of your child developing MS, assuming the father does not also have MS, is low, being in the region of 2 per cent (1 in 50). All things considered, having MS is not a reason for deciding not to have children.

I would love some more children but am worried I won't be able to cope with a new baby as well as my daughter who is now three. What do you advise?

As discussed above, there are no medical reasons why you shouldn't have as many children as you want. Some people find that MS makes them much more tired and this can make coping with young children more difficult. However, this can be managed by both tackling the fatigue itself (see the section on 'Fatigue' in Chapter 14) and by ensuring that you involve friends and family in helping out to make sure you get enough rest.

If there are any particular issues that are concerning you, have a chat with your neurologist, MS nurse or GP.

BREASTFEEDING

What about breastfeeding? Will it have any effect on my MS?

There is no proven effect, either good or bad, of breastfeeding on MS. However, breastfeeding is widely known to be good for babies, as well as for the mother-baby bonding process – so try to do it if you can even if for only a few weeks. Your midwife and health visitor are there to support you if needed. If you were on a disease-modifying drug before you got pregnant, it is probably best to delay restarting treatment until you have finished breastfeeding.

Can I take steroids or disease-modifying drugs if I am breastfeeding?

It is not known whether beta-interferon (Avonex, Betaferon, Extavia, Rebif 22/44), glatiramer acetate (Copaxone) or natalizumab (Tysabri) are excreted in breast milk and so their use in nursing mothers is not generally recommended. If you have a bad relapse while breast-feeding, and you need treatment with high dose steroids, it is usually recommended that you pump and discard any breastmilk produced for a few hours after each dose of medication.

I want to breastfeed but I don't feel confident. Is there anything I can do to make things easier?

Remember to discuss your wishes and concerns regarding breast-feeding with your MS nurse and midwife as early as possible. They will be able to give you advice regarding positioning the baby, especially if you have weakness or numbness in your arms. You may be able to feed your baby lying down on your side, with your baby on the floor, to conserve energy.

Managing fatigue effectively is also important. Remember it is important to look after yourself and ensure that you eat regularly. You may be able to express milk for your partner to assist with some of the night feeds which will help with the lack of sleep! Your partner could bring your baby to you to feed, allowing you to maximise your rest. Alternatively, your partner may perform some of your other domestic responsibilities to allow you to focus on your baby.

20 | Living with MS

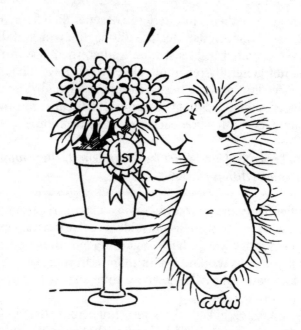

Some of the key issues affecting people with MS and their families concern practical problems of managing employment, housing, insurance and other financial issues, exercise, leisure and holidays, dealing with social services, as well as investigating possibilities for respite and long-term care in MS.

EMPLOYMENT AND MS

Can I do my job now that I have been diagnosed with MS?

This depends on your job and the symptoms you are experiencing, but hopefully the answer will be yes. The majority of people diagnosed with MS do continue to work for many years after receiving their diagnosis although high numbers of people with MS do have to retire earlier than they would perhaps choose.

If your job is particularly physical in nature or may be dangerous for someone with MS (for example lots of high ladder work or driving a heavy goods vehicle) then you may need to look for other work options. Employers are bound by the Disability Discrimination Act to support you in continuing to work in your current role as long as possible or to help you in finding alternative roles within the company if appropriate.

We do advise people to continue working for as long as they feel able to. Work provides so many of us with structure, and with social contact, with friends and colleagues as well as helping us define our sense of self. That said, some people do not enjoy work and much prefer to leave and retrain or take ill health retirement, depending on individual circumstances. This can be a very positive move: we have known several people who have left their jobs after been given a diagnosis of MS who have gone on to retrain or start their own business and are now much happier than they were before they knew they had MS. MS can open doors as well as shutting them sometimes.

Now that I have been diagnosed with MS, do I have to tell my employer?

If you are already employed when you receive your diagnosis, you are not legally bound to tell your employer although you will probably find it much easier if you do so. Once your employer is aware of your diagnosis, they are bound by the Disability Discrimination Act (DDA) to support you and to help enable you to carry out your job as easily as you can. This may mean ensuring you are based on the ground floor or within reach of the toilets, or it may mean that your employer provides you with an air conditioning unit or allows you to work more flexibly or from home. You do not need to tell colleagues if you do not wish them to know.

If you apply for a new job once you have been diagnosed with MS, you are obliged to answer truthfully any health-related questions. In practice, this is likely to mean telling them your diagnosis. Again, the Disability Discrimination Act (DDA) should prevent any selection bias purely on the grounds of your diagnosis.

I understand that the provisions of the Disability Discrimination Act (1995) apply to many aspects of employment for people with disabilities. How might they affect someone with MS?

The Disability Discrimination Act (DDA) was extended in 2005 and now provides protection for people with MS from diagnosis onwards, regardless of the symptoms they experience. This means that employers must provide reasonable support for anyone with MS in their company, in order to allow them to continue in their role or to look at other roles within the company which may be more suitable.

The Disability Discrimination Act also means that shops and services have a duty to ensure they are accessible to people with disabilities.

Can I be sacked because I have MS? What legal protection is there for someone in my position?

You cannot be sacked just because you have MS. The Disability Discrimination Act covers anyone with a diagnosis of MS and means that a company has to make all reasonable adjustments to retain you within the workforce. If you are still unable to fulfil your duties because of the problems you are having due to your MS, then alternative roles or the option of ill-health retirement should be discussed.

I am finding it rather difficult to find a job that I can do now that my MS has become more severe. What do you suggest I do?

This can be a big problem, and many people find that the combination of fatigue and cognitive problems alone can make it very difficult to work. Estimates vary as to how many people with MS are unable to work, but some studies put this as high as 80 per cent (4 out of 5 people). Some people are able to resolve this by working for themselves. This allows them to work much more flexibly, taking on as much or as little work as they can manage, and letting them pace their work to fit the way they are feeling. Unfortunately, the majority of people with MS are not in a position where this is an option, and most people with severe MS are unable to work.

However, there are people and organisations that can help. One of these is Job Centre Plus which provides help and advice for people with all sorts of health problems in finding employment. There are also a number of different voluntary sector agencies that can help, and it is worth looking locally to see what other help is available. Your occupational therapist or MS nurse may be able to point you in the right direction.

If you are unable to find a post that suits you, it is worth considering voluntary work. Many people find this very enjoyable. Just a couple of hours a week may be enough to get you out of the house and give you an opportunity to meet others. It also helps you continue to contribute to society which has a positive effect on your self-esteem.

If I apply for a new job, am I obliged to tell my prospective employers about my MS?

If you are asked a direct question about your health or whether you have a disability or long-term illness, then you do have to declare your diagnosis. This should be for the best as the Disability Discrimination Act prevents employers discriminating against anyone with a disability and it also means that you will be able to access any additional support you may need as soon as you start your new job. If you don't declare your diagnosis when asked, and your employers later find out you have MS, they are within their rights to dismiss you. So it does pay to be open with employers from the start.

Should I tell my colleagues about my MS?

This is a common question, the answer to which really depends very much on individual circumstances. As a rule of thumb, we would advise people to share their diagnosis of MS, and some of the ways this affects them, with their colleagues. The majority of people find their colleagues are then much more understanding, helpful and supportive than they may have been otherwise. Unfortunately, not everyone works alongside people they feel they can confide in, and this does have to be an individual decision. It is important, however, that someone at work is aware of your condition. Even if you can't talk to your colleagues about it, you should discuss your MS with either your line manager or their manager, to ensure that your employer is aware you have MS and that you are not under any undue pressure, or asked to take on any roles which might be unreasonably difficult for you. Both the MS Society and the MS Trust produce useful information leaflets that address this issue in more detail.

SOCIAL LIFE

Since I have been diagnosed with MS, I've given up many interests that I had before, and this seems to make me even more preoccupied with my condition. My doctor and many of my friends urge me to take up my interests again. What do you think?

It is a good thing you have been talking to people about this and have discussed it with your doctor. It is possible you may be a little depressed and it is important to talk to others about how you are feeling.

It would certainly be a good idea to take up take up some of the interests you had before and even to look for new things that may be of interest to you too. If there is something you would like to take up again, but are finding it difficult for any reason, do discuss this with your occupational therapist or MS nurse, as they may well have useful suggestions. An occupational therapist or MS nurse may also be able to tell you about other options available to you locally which you may find interesting and which would motivate you to get out and meet some new people. Making the effort to take up hobbies and interests again can feel very hard at first, but do persevere. Once you have pushed yourself to make the initial effort, it will get much easier. You will be surprised how much better you feel once you have something to think about other than your MS.

I am worried about doing active things like sports or gardening, because the MS is beginning to affect my mobility. Will these activities harm me?

No – do continue to keep active and pursue your interests for as long as you can. You may find that you are able to do less gardening or sports before needing to rest, however, and you may find that you need to make slight changes to the way you approach things. For example, you may find you need to take a seat out with you in the garden to use when weeding, or that you are better planting things in raised beds, or that using more pots and containers makes it easier for you to reach and tend to your plants. Alternatively, you may find that you need to change the sorts of machines you use in the gym, or switch to swimming rather than cycling. But there is almost always something you can do to get round any problems you are having. So long as you are not so tired that you are wiped out for hours afterwards, or so unsteady that you are at real risk of hurting yourself, then staying active – doing something you enjoy – can only be helpful.

My husband and I like going out to places like the theatre and cinema, or stately homes and gardens, but my MS has reduced my mobility and I have to use a wheelchair on some occasions. We have found before that wheelchair access is often difficult, and sometimes impossible. What should we do?

The Disability Discrimination Act now puts the onus on all public places, facilities and services to do all they reasonably can to ensure anyone with a disability can access their premises and other services. Certainly, places like cinemas and theatres should be accessible to you and your wheelchair. If you phone them beforehand they will be able to explain their facilities and discuss with you any special needs you both may have. In addition, cinemas and theatres often have concessionary offers for people visiting with a wheelchair user.

Unfortunately, gaining access to stately homes, gardens and other places of historical interest may be more difficult, as their age and design can make it impossible to fit the necessary adaptations. Do contact wherever you are planning to visit before you go in order to find out about the situation in advance. Very often, at least part of the house and gardens will be wheelchair accessible, or staff may be able to come up with other ways round the problem and will often go out of their way to help if they can. The National Trust, for instance, makes sure that all its properties have adapted WCs and enable access for wheelchair users as far as the limitations of the properties will allow. There are also a number of websites (see the list at the back of this book) which provide information about locally accessible venues for people with disabilities.

We have found holidays increasingly difficult because my husband has MS, and we have not had a proper holiday for a long time. Are there special sources of help or advice you could suggest?

This can be a real problem, and it is often difficult to rely on the information about accessibility provided in some holiday brochures. A grab rail in the toilet does not necessarily mean a room is 'disabled friendly'!

The best way to find somewhere to stay is by word of mouth – talk to others with MS if you can or approach your local branch of the MS Society to see whether they have any suggestions. The MS Society also has information about suitable holidays, so have a look at their website or contact their helpline. If you use the Internet, there are a number of different websites providing useful information (see Appendix 1). There is also helpful information about travelling with MS.

Once you think you have found somewhere you would like to stay, do contact the people who run the place before booking and ask specific questions relating to your particular needs. Their idea of a room suitable for use by someone with MS and what you actually need may be very different. It may also be worth discussing this with your social worker or MS nurse – particularly if you have carers coming in when you are at home or use specialised equipment such as hoists. Your social worker or MS nurse will be able to help you make sure you have the necessary equipment and help that you need in place while you are away. Your MS nurse can also help if you are worried about managing any particular symptoms (such as bladder problems or spasms) that may cause problems while you are travelling or away.

Holidays are meant to be fun, and with a little planning yours can be too. Enjoy!

FINANCES

This section deals with some very complicated issues. This is not only because people's circumstances vary, but because the rules and regulations governing eligibility to benefits, pensions and so on, are themselves complex and appear to change frequently. It is very important that, in addition to taking note of the points made below, you consult other sources of information. Choices that you may make about continuing or leaving work, or about benefits and pensions, may have long-lasting consequences, so it is important to think them through carefully after seeking impartial advice.

Sources of information include:

- *Disability Rights Handbook*, published by the Disability Alliance (see Appendix 2);
- Department for Work and Pensions;
- Citizens' Advice;
- Welfare Rights Office
- Your local authority and the MS Society's Welfare Rights Adviser.

Financial help for drivers is discussed in Chapter 15, in the section on Driving.

I have MS. Am I entitled to any help while I am still working?

The benefits system is complex and changes quite frequently. There are benefits for which some people are eligible to claim when they are working though this depends on the problems you have as a result of your MS and the amount of work you are doing. The best people to contact for advice on your particular circumstances, and who can help you apply for any benefits you are eligible for, would be your local Citizens Advice Bureau or Welfare Rights Office. There are contact details for the main offices of these organisations in Appendix 1, or you can find details of your local offices in the phone book.

I have had increasing problems with sickness due to MS over the last few months, and thus have had to take a lot of time off work. What benefits might I be eligible for?

Again this is a complicated area and you should seek advice from an organisation such as Citizens Advice or the local Welfare Rights Office. Generally speaking, however, employers are bound to pay Statutory Sick Pay to any employee who has been off work for four days or more, for up to 28 weeks. You may also be eligible for Income Support if you are on a low income. If you are off sick for longer than 28 weeks, you may be eligible for Employment and Support Allowance, which replaced Incapacity Benefit from October 2008. This provides an income for people currently unable to work and, at the same time, provides support and help to enable people to return to work if they are able to do so.

If I decide to stop working completely, what are likely to be the financial consequences, and what benefits will I get?

This depends very much on your individual circumstances. Some people are in a relatively good financial position and are able to claim a pension from their employers on the grounds of ill-health retirement. If you belong to a pension scheme, it is important that you explore this option further with your employers and/or the pension company.

People who are unable to work will initially be able to claim Employment and Support Allowance. As part of this, you will be assessed for your ability to return to work and given any help you need to achieve this goal. If you are deemed to be unable to work, you will then be eligible to receive Support Allowance for as long as you require it. If you are on a low income, you may also be eligible for Income Support. Your local Welfare Rights Office or Citizens Advice will be able to give you individual advice and support with any claims you may need to make.

What is the Disability Living Allowance and who can claim it?

The Disability Living Allowance (or DLA) is available to anyone under the age of 65 years of age who has difficulty walking and/or needs help to care for themselves. The DLA is made up of two components known as 'Care' and 'Mobility'. Some people may be eligible for both, while others will be eligible just for one of the components. Mobility Allowance is payable to people who are unable to walk or who have significant difficulties walking, while the Care component is payable to people who need help to look after themselves.

If you are not sure whether or not to make a claim for Disability Living Allowance, discuss this with your social worker, MS nurse, GP or another health or social care professional who knows you.

Do I have to tell my insurance company that I have MS?

If you are taking out new insurance and your insurance company asks any questions about your health and any medical tests or scans you have had, you must answer them honestly (of course) or you will find the insurance is not valid. The MS Society (see Appendix 1) can help if you have problems finding insurance, although this isn't usually a problem.

If you have existing insurance that you are concerned about when you are diagnosed, you should check your policy booklet for advice or contact the MS Society helpline. How much you should tell a company with which you have an existing policy will depend very much on the type of insurance policy you have, as well as on your individual circumstances.

Do mortgage lenders and insurance companies discriminate against people who have MS?

Mortgage lenders and insurance companies should base their rates and insurance deals on your individual circumstances, in the same way as they would with any other customer. They are forbidden by law to discriminate against you purely on the basis of your diagnosis. If you have any difficulties finding insurance or a mortgage to suit your needs, the MS Society helpline can offer information and advice.

Am I entitled to free prescriptions?

If you live in England, unfortunately, a diagnosis of MS does not automatically entitle you to free prescriptions, although the MS Society and MS Trust are lobbying hard to change this. You are entitled to free prescriptions if you are under 19 and in full time education, over 60, receiving Income Support or cannot leave the house without help. In the latter case you need to obtain form FP92A from your GP and send it to the prescription pricing authority.

If you live in Scotland or Wales and are registered with a Welsh or Scottish GP, your prescriptions will be free. Free prescriptions for all should be introduced into Northern Ireland by 2010.

Can I also claim for eye and dental care costs?

You are only entitled to free dental and eye care if you are under 19 and in full time education, over 60, pregnant or have had a child within the last 12 months, or are receiving Income Support. You are also entitled to free eye tests if you have diabetes, are registered blind or partially sighted, or have been diagnosed as having glaucoma or have a first degree relative with glaucoma and are over 40.

These regulations are complicated and do change from time to time so do check with your GP, pharmacist, dentist or optician before starting treatment.

SUPPORT

I am going to have a 'Needs Assessment'. What will this involve?

A Needs Assessment is carried out by social services to determine what care services you may require. It will involve your social worker visiting you at home and talking with you and your partner (or main carer) to identify the main tasks during the day with which you need help, and to discuss the sort of help they can offer. It is then up to you to decide with the social worker what package of care would best suit your needs.

What kinds of services might be available following a Needs Assessment and care plan?

Once you have been seen by a social worker and had a Needs Assessment, you will be offered different options. The most common sort of help available is from carers from a care agency who come in and help out with personal needs such as helping you get up in the morning, washed and dressed, or helping you get to bed at night. These carers can also come in during the day if you need help getting your meals or getting to the toilet, but they cannot help out with, for example, housework or shopping – only with personal care. The social worker may also discuss with you and your partner/carer options including respite care or attendance at a day centre once or twice during the week. This would give you both a bit of a break, and to help you get out of the house and meet new people.

There may also be other schemes operating locally such as Crossroads or Independent Living which your social worker can provide to give you and your partner/carer more flexibility in the way you decide to structure your week.

In most areas, another alternative known as Direct Payments is available.

So what are Direct Payments and how do they work?

For Direct Payments to be awarded, your social worker will first undertake a Needs Assessment in order, as described above, to determine the total amount of care you need each week. This is then converted into a sum of money which you can use to employ someone directly to undertake the care you need. This is a much more complex process as you become the employer and have to recruit your carers yourself and then manage their salary, national insurance and holiday pay. However, some people much prefer the flexibility this system provides as they are able to choose who cares for them and when the care is given, rather than being tied to the staff and times an agency provides.

If you think you may be interested in pursuing Direct Payments, you should discuss this with your social worker and explore the advantages and disadvantages relevant to your particular circumstances. It won't be the best option for everyone.

I care for my wife. Can I be assessed for my needs?

Yes, you can. Since the Carers Act in 1995, carers have been entitled to a Needs Assessment. You can ask to see a social worker in your own right, even if your wife does not want to see one. The social worker will discuss with you any concerns and problems you may be having and suggest options that are available to help make things easier for you both.

My wife has MS. We have got to the point where she cannot really get up the stairs any more. What are our options for staying on in our home, or should we move?

This is always a difficult time and can mean complete reorganisation of the way you live your lives and use your home. If you are happy otherwise with where you are living, you should contact an occupational therapist who can come and see you both at home and discuss the various options available. You can either contact an occupational therapist directly yourself, or ask another health or social care professional to refer you.

Some people are able to manage with a stair lift, although not all authorities will fit stair lifts as they can become unsafe if the person with MS is unable to transfer or has particular problems with balance while sitting. Another option is to have a through floor lift fitted – these are much less obtrusive than they sound and can be sent up (or down) out of the way when not required. A third option, which people often take up, is to have an extension built on the house or to have the garage converted into a downstairs bedroom with an en-suite toilet and bathroom. None of these options are cheap – your occupational therapist will be able to talk through the financial implications with you. Grants are available for all or some of the necessary funding, though these are means-tested.

As you say, the alternative is to move house. So the decision as to whether to have your current home adapted or whether to move house is inevitably a very individual one. Before making this decision, do talk to your occupational therapist and discuss the available options with him or her. Look around at suitable properties in the area you would like to live in, think hard about the financial implications of moving and discuss all the options with friends and family. You also need to think about whether you can get a house near enough to your current support networks to enable you to continue seeing your friends and family members as much as before. This is a major decision for you both and not one which you should rush.

> *I look after my husband and have been told that I can have*
> *respite care. What exactly does this mean?*

Respite care can make a huge difference to both of you. This involves making arrangements for your husband to stay else-where for a period of time to allow both of you to have a break. Respite care centres vary widely depending on local resources. The MS Society has its own specialist respite care centres which are available (though they do tend to get booked up quickly!) and also has a preferred provider scheme by which respite centres are identified which are considered to be able to give high levels of care to people with MS.

Respite care can sometimes be arranged in your local Nursing Home or Residential Home, and you and your husband will be able to visit any local centres before deciding whether to take up the offer of respite care.

Deciding to accept respite care can be very difficult for some, and it is sometimes the case that the care available will not be at the same high levels you are able to give your husband at home. However, it is important that you try to find somewhere that is acceptable, as respite care can make a huge difference to you both – and particularly to you as the carer. It will allow you time to rest and recharge your batteries, and spend some time doing things for yourself. It may feel very strange to put yourself first for a change but if you are not well and strong you won't be able to look after your husband as you would like, despite your best efforts. Respite care helps to keep you well and strong.

21 | You and your family

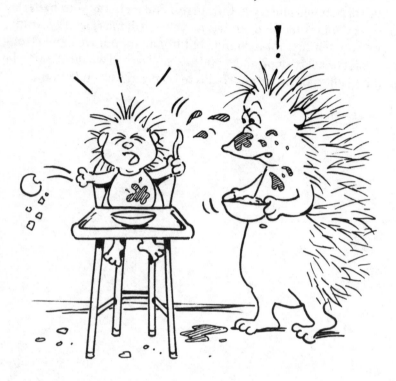

RELATIONSHIPS WITH PARTNERS

Managing relationships with partners is difficult even without the presence of MS.

How much MS itself affects such relationships is always hard to judge precisely, because of the many different kinds of relationships that exist between two people. Of course, MS does bring complications of its own, sometimes major ones that have to be dealt with, but it often highlights the positive and the negative aspects of relationships which were already there.

With my MS everything seems to be so uncertain from day to day, even from minute to minute. My husband doesn't really understand. Is there anything we can do to help each other?

As you imply, the uncertainties linked with MS are difficult to manage for both of you. On one hand, the 'hidden' symptoms of MS such as fatigue and continence problems, can appear at any time, thus placing you in a situation where you may not be able to plan even more than a few minutes ahead in relation to your daily activities. On the other hand, your life with MS requires planning to ensure that when you do things, you can make the best possible arrangements to ensure that you can do them well. All this can be very frustrating.

Although the longer term future with MS is uncertain, the key daily problem for many people is managing their fatigue. As we have noted in Chapter 14, there are many things you can do to tackle your fatigue. It is also possible to increase your stamina a little through careful exercise: your physiotherapist and/or MS nurse should be able to give you some individual advice about the best way to approach this. Involving your husband in this may help.

The main strategy should be to get to know your own daily rhythms and events. The key thing as far as your husband is concerned is to try and get him to appreciate that the variability in your symptoms is not your fault or under your direct control. This is sometimes difficult, for even those people who know you well may feel sometimes that, when you say you are too tired to do something you have planned, you are 'putting it on'. It might help if your husband were to read a bit more about MS (perhaps this book), or to discuss this issue with your occupational therapist, MS nurse, neurologist or another health professional who knows the effects of MS well. He should then be able to see that the uncertainties and changes in your symptoms are due to the MS and that you are every bit as frustrated as he is about them.

We know that, in some families, the problems associated with MS become such a major focus that relationships can break down. It is important to work out ways of sharing or developing other mutual interests involving less physical activity perhaps. Tell your husband about services that are available for 'carers' (see the section later in this chapter on *Being a carer*) so that he knows he is not alone in his feelings and problems.

> *I suppose you could say I've always been a 'houseproud' person, and wanted to make a good home for my husband and myself. I really feel our relationship is now in difficulties because, with my MS, I can't keep the house going as I should. What should I do?*

Relationships are built on all kinds of different things. However, despite modern attitudes, looking after the home well is still something which many women, and often their partners, feel is important. It may be difficult to deal with a situation where it becomes hard for you to do this, but it would be very unusual for a relationship to be built only on looking after the home well – there will be other things that you like and share in common.

Housework is often seen by women as something which reflects personally on them and by which they feel the rest of the world judges them – although in practice very few people will even notice whether or not you have managed to clean up today or whether you have changed the beds, for example (and if they do then point them in the direction of the vacuum cleaner). Letting go of housework so that you can spend more time doing things that are important to both of you can be very hard but is worth doing. Divide the housework up into chunks which can be done in stages over the week, and ask for help. Make sure you get the rest of the family involved and apportion household tasks. Another option worth considering is to employ a cleaner for just a few hours a week who can help with the particularly heavy tasks or can do the ironing or change the beds – things which you may find very difficult or tiring yourself but which need to be done.

If you continue to have difficulties with this and certainly if you feel your relationship is suffering as a result, then talk to your MS nurse, GP or other health professional. There may be aids or equipment which could help you manage the housework more easily or other suggestions pertinent to your individual circumstances which your MS nurse can discuss with you.

Both my partner and I have always looked after ourselves, and people say what an attractive couple we make. But I really am worried that the MS will ruin our relationship.

MS often affects people when they are young. They may worry that things like physical appearance, which younger people value more, will be totally lost. Apart from some unusual situations when the MS proceeds very rapidly, it is likely to be some time before there are very visible long-term bodily effects. In the longer term, of course, everyone with or without MS has to adjust to the effects of ageing! As with any situation it is important to keep talking to each other – be honest about how you are feeling, your worries and concerns, and hopefully you can then work through these together rather than dealing with your worries alone. Dealing with the problems that MS brings can often bring couples closer together and strengthen relationships.

RELATIONSHIPS WITH CHILDREN

My 6-year-old girl says she is worried that she might get MS, now that she has seen her mummy with the condition. What do I say to her?

Although children may worry about this, their anxiety may not emerge explicitly in family discussions. In Chapter 3, we talk about the inherited component of MS. The risk is very small so you should be very reassuring. You should also reassure your daughter on another point, that MS is not 'catching' or contagious. Sometimes children feel anything that is, in their experience, out of the ordinary, may be 'catching', largely because so many adult discussions with children about health, talk about problems of 'catching' illnesses from other people – both from adults and children. A couple of very useful booklets produced by the MS Society and the MS Trust (details of both organisations are in Appendix 1) aimed at young children are available, and you may find these useful for talking through some of the worries your daughter has. The best approach is usually to be led by your daughter and just be as open, honest and as matter of fact with her as you can, answering her questions as they arise. Children often cope much better than we expect them to and are much more accepting of problems caused by MS than most adults.

At first I was concerned about the possibility of passing on my MS to my children. Now my main concern is being able to bring them up as I should. Will I be able to do this properly?

Of course it depends what you mean by 'properly'! Most future parents are very committed to wanting the best for their child, and have clear views about what they want to avoid as well as how they want to be as parents. It is quite right that they have those ambitions, but most parents find, in practice, that their world with children is more complicated, less predictable and less easy to manage than planned: relationships between partners break down; jobs change or are lost and money can be tight, so compromises have to be made. In addition, children, as most parents find, have minds and wishes of their own!

Having MS, with the various problems it might bring in parenting, is just one factor among many that may affect the bringing up of children. Do not feel that, without the MS, parenting of children would somehow be easy, as having young children is a major physical burden in terms of managing their hour-to-hour activities, feeding, wayward sleeping patterns and so on. For the early years of a child's life, it is important, as it would be for all people, to think through daily activities with your partner, and also with other family members if possible, to enable you to feel that the burden of daily child care activities is not going to rest entirely on you. Such support in the end may make the difference between feeling child care is an almost impossibly demanding activity, and feeling that it is at the very least tolerable, and hopefully very rewarding.

I have two young children who are not yet at school. How much should I tell them about my MS?

Many parents worry about when and how to tell their children that they have MS. Such a view is often based on a misunderstanding of what a child, even a very young one, is likely to have observed, or even to have understood. Children are very acute observers, and almost certainly will have picked up on any anxieties – about MS as well as other things – some time before you think they have. They may not know exactly what 'MS' is, but will probably already be aware that mummy or daddy may find difficulties in doing some things, or that there are heated (or hushed) discussions about other things to do with everyday life.

In such a situation, when the opportunity arises, perhaps when you are trying to do a particularly difficult task, then a matter-of-fact, non-technical and brief explanation as to how the difficulty has arisen will be helpful, however young the children are. Over time, these explanations can be elaborated. The key thing is to treat the MS, as almost certainly you do yourself, as an everyday issue, rather than one with mountainous implications for the future, which may upset your children.

Children may well ask questions themselves such as 'Why did you nearly fall over then?' or 'Why are you wobbly?' or 'Why are you walking with a stick?' If this happens, you should answer, matter of factly and as honestly as you can, by talking, for example, about your illness as something which means that your legs don't always move as well as they should, because messages to your leg muscles from your brain don't always get through. This makes you wobbly and you have to use a stick (or wheelchair) to help you. You can say more about MS itself, or indeed about other symptoms, on other occasions, or when they ask for more detail. An honest and matter of fact approach often works best.

Although parents may try, understandably, to protect their children from what the parents see as the disturbing aspects of MS, young children may think that there is a major family secret not being discussed with them, and which is very threatening – precisely because it is not talked through. Fears might include the early death of the parent with MS, or indeed their own deaths. You should be reassuring about both of these issues.

To be generally reassuring, talk about the MS with your children as though it is a part – although only a part – of their lives, as it is of yours. Explain things as each situation arises, especially when children themselves are curious or ask questions. If children feel you are being honest in responding to their questions or concerns, both you and they are less likely to have problems later. The booklets produced by the MS Society and MS Trust aimed at explaining MS to young and teenage children can also be very useful and may be a way of broaching the subject if this has become difficult.

My 12-year-old son seems to feel that he is responsible for my MS, and keeps on worrying about us looking after him. He thinks he is a burden on us. How can I reassure him?

Many children, particularly those who are under pressure, may feel that they are to blame in some way for the MS, perhaps by having been 'naughty' in the past. They often don't explicitly say this to their parents – at least in your case you are aware of your son's feelings. Be reassuring about this point, and ensure that your son is aware that, whatever he may or may not have done, this had no bearing on your MS. Of course, some mothers may have (mistakenly) blamed their MS itself, or some of its symptoms, on a pregnancy and the associated childbirth – it is possible that this feeling has been picked up by a child.

The fact that your son feels he is a burden on you needs some mutual discussion, to ascertain why he feels this way, and how best to manage these feelings. Often – to parents' surprise – children do feel as responsible for their parents, as their parents feel responsible for them. This is particularly likely if there appears to be some problem (such as long-term illness) which is causing difficulties in their family. Allow your son to express his concern for you, and show your appreciation of that concern, but also reassure him that he is *not* a burden on you in the way he thinks, and is loved for being himself. Try to agree some small ways in which he can help – by doing some specific jobs in the house, for example. This can help him feel that he is contributing to the family.

> *My daughter is in her final A level year in her sixth form college, and I assumed that she would go to university – which we should like her to do. However, although she applied, and has already obtained a place at a university several hours' journey from our home, she now tells me that she doesn't want to go, and at the same time, says how worried she is about me.*

There could be several reasons for this. Although many young people like your daughter do go to university, others have different plans – at least immediately after they have left school – and will take up a job without going to university, or perhaps postpone their entry until a little later in life. As universities and colleges are now much more geared to admitting and supporting what they describe as 'mature' students, going to university later in life should not prove a major problem from that point of view.

However, as your daughter has linked her wish that she now doesn't want to go to university with her concern for you, it does seem that there may be issues here to do with your MS. It is important to tell her that you want her to go to university, without putting undue pressure on her. You need to reassure her that you do not think it is her role, or her duty to look after you. At the same time, indicate how you propose to deal with any further disability that may develop – this will reassure her that you have been thinking about such issues yourself. She may be worried also about your (and her) financial position at university. Be as reassuring as you can, and perhaps seek advice yourself about likely financial issues, to be better informed yourself before speaking to her. The main aim here is to give as much acknowledgement as possible to her views, ambitions and concerns, and to indicate that her priorities are as important as those of others in the family.

I am very concerned at my situation. My husband left me three years ago and, as my MS has got worse, I have become very dependent on my 14-year-old daughter to help me with all kinds of things, such as washing me and helping me to the toilet.

The issue of 'young carers' is one which has come to public attention more and more over the past few years. It is a complex issue. People who do not know your situation might think that your daughter is 'losing her childhood or early adolescence' and wish to have her removed from the tasks that you describe, and her general caring role, immediately. Such an immediate reaction might produce an even more difficult situation. It is important to try to achieve a balanced view of how to proceed.

The key issue is how children can help but still ensure their own futures through doing well in formal education, and through play and leisure in their own time. In the first instance, you should contact your local Adult Disability team within Social Services (the number should be in your phone book – if not your GP's surgery or local Council offices will be able to give you the contact number). Once you have requested an assessment, a social worker will come and see you at home and talk to you about the problems you are having and discuss the different types of help they can offer.

Many people have carers who come in between once and four times a day to help with personal cares such as washing and dressing which may take some of the pressure off your daughter. It is important to be aware of all the options open to you and your daughter so that you can then make an informed decision about which option would best suit your needs.

Carers' groups (listed in Appendix 1) now have specific advice and resources for young carers. These can be an excellent source of support for your daughter and often run a range of different activities with other children in similar situations which most young people find a lot of fun.

My son, who is now 15, doesn't do a thing in the house or help me. He wants to go out with his friends all the time, many of whom we don't approve. My wife and I have tried hard to bring him up well, but we are now in despair about him.

We hear many parents saying the same thing as you, even without MS in the family! Bringing up children, and particularly teenagers, is a problem for any family. It is difficult to know how much your son has reacted to your MS, or whether there are other factors involved. However, the early and mid-teen years are when young people of both sexes are beginning to assert their independence from their family – often generating difficult and fraught family relationships. This is a necessary part of 'growing up', which family members, and particularly parents, may have difficulty acknowledging. Exactly what effects the addition of MS have in any individual family setting is difficult to judge.

It may be that he is just 'being a teenager', or he may feel too much pressure to stay at home and help which will curb his freedom even more. Although you are undoubtedly under considerable pressure yourself, the only way this is likely to be resolved is through patience and tolerance. You could seek some informal advice and support from other parents in a similar situation, for example, in your local MS Society branch, or consult your doctor about a possible referral for family therapy where all the members of the family could talk through the situation and consider ways forward.

> *As a man with MS I am really concerned about my role in disciplining my children. I am not very mobile at the moment, but I want them to know that I am still 'in charge'.*

The issue of disciplining children is a tricky and difficult one for parents with MS, and particularly for fathers. There are different styles of discipline, some more forceful and direct than others. The more effective your expertise in negotiation and communication, the less likely it will be that you have to resort to direct discipline of a kind that requires you to raise your voice or move quickly.

Because some fathers cannot join in with physical games and activities, particularly with sons, they try to assert their authority in other ways. However, remember that children are very adaptable. You might have a good knowledge of sport, or you could participate in other things in which they are interested. All children need to see where the boundaries lie, but if the boundaries are always drawn in a fiercely robust and negative rather than positive way, then you may be storing up some problems for the future. Challenging behaviour may be related to their underlying fears about you and your MS, and this may require quite a different response.

Don't forget that parenting, including disciplining children, should be undertaken with the help of others, including partners and family members. Don't feel that you have to do it all on your own.

> *I feel exhausted when my children come home from school. They want my attention, and want to show me things and involve me in all the things they do – but often I just haven't the energy.*

Fatigue associated with MS is often a problem, and as we have noted in Chapter 14, a combination of a careful assessment of your own daily patterns of fatigue, and possibly some medication from your doctor or MS nurse, will help you plan the day a bit better, so that you can include the children more in your activities.

Other mothers with MS usually deal with these problems by pacing activities during the earlier part of the day. You can then rest before the children come home from school. If you are working outside the home, then again it is important, if you can, to schedule a time where you can relax and rest before giving your attention to your children. Try to discuss the problem with your children, so that they are aware that you want to find a way in which you can have regular and dedicated time together. You could perhaps put together a combination of 'time slots' with slightly less demanding activities. This may provide other benefits as well, in the form of closer ties with your children, and their understanding of you and your difficulties.

> *Once or twice my daughter – who is now 11 years old – has been a little late for school because I haven't been able to get everything ready for her in the morning, and from time to time she has had to help me. Should I let the school know about my MS?*

In most circumstances it is important that you do so. You do not say, and maybe you do not know, what reasons your daughter has given to the school when she has been late. As schools are becoming more concerned about pupils' punctuality, it is a good idea to let at least her class teacher know about your situation. The school may arrange a meeting with her teacher, so that any questions or concerns that the teacher may have about MS, as well as any consequences for your daughter, could be discussed. You can address the issue of occasional lateness, and you will be also reassured that the teacher understands MS and its effects more accurately. If you can establish a good and collaborative relationship with your daughter's main class or form teacher, it is likely that you will all benefit. Your daughter will probably not want to be seen by her peers or her teachers as someone who is 'very different' from others in her class, and so you should be sensitive to her worries about how these discussions are handled at the school.

BEING A CARER

I am really annoyed with the word 'carer' when it's applied to me. I suppose I am doing the caring, but he's my husband and I'm not just a carer!

Some people do have negative feelings about the word 'carer' – they feel like a 'one-dimensional' person, that it implies they have no life or interests of their own and that it undermines in some way the caring you want to do for your husband as his wife. On the other hand, others feel that being called a 'carer' is much more positive, for it recognises the many things that you do for the person with MS, which can otherwise be just taken for granted. Of course, increasingly there are services and support targeted at 'carers'. You should take advantage of those services, even if it means, for these purposes, that you are considered a carer.

It is very important that everybody, from friends to professionals, recognises that your relationship with your husband is much more complex than caring alone, and that you have your own interests, ideas and concerns. Make sure that you have time to yourself so that you can 'recharge your batteries' outside the daily and often onerous demands of being a carer and wife.

I really feel my life is a constant battle for services and support for my wife. Nothing seems easy or simple to obtain.

This is a very common complaint by family members of people with MS. Part of the problem is often that there seems to be no central source of information which can be used to access those services that you need, now and possibly later. You will need to experiment to find out what is the best source in your area.

The Internet is a great source of information nowadays and well worth exploring if you have access to it. The MS Society and MS Trust both have maps on their websites giving some information about local services and can certainly let you know who the local neurologist and MS nurse are. The local MS Society branch will also be able to give you information about available local services.

Once you have identified your MS nurse, it is always worth contacting him or her. MS nurses are usually not only be able to tell you which services can help, but are also able to liaise with the different services, if required. Your GP's surgery and your local library can also be useful sources of information – particularly if you are unable to access or use the Internet.

22 | Other relationships

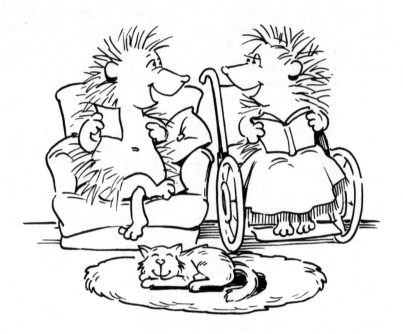

Dealing with relationships with people outside your immediate circle of close friends and family can be like crossing a minefield. Who should you tell and how? Do you have to tell anyone? How can you best develop a useful relationship with the different health professionals with whom you will inevitably come into contact? In this final chapter we explore some of these issues and suggest ways in which you can ensure that MS does not impact too much on other relationships in your life.

RELATIONSHIPS WITH FRIENDS

My friends often tell me how well I look – even when I'm feeling bad – and it's even worse when I am having a really bad day and using my wheelchair. I sometimes hear whispers like 'Why is he in a wheelchair? He looks OK'. What can I do?

Many of the symptoms of MS are so called 'invisible' – problems such as pain, fatigue, limb weakness, even bladder and bowel problems are not evident to other people in the same way that a broken leg or operation scar can be. People tend to be able to relate to these more familiar problems in a way they usually find much more difficult with something like MS, which they may not understand.

You should consider their comments as a compliment – that at least you do look well – even though you may not feel it all the time. And take the opportunity to help them understand a bit more about what it feels like to live with MS. If you are feeling up to it perhaps you can make a joke of it next time they comment. Let them know you have heard, tell them that you wish you felt as well as you look and explain a little about how you feel.

Since I have had MS, I feel it is very difficult to make friends. I'm beginning to feel that the future is looking bleak socially as well as physically.

You are still, in many ways, the same person as you were before the MS. Although the MS has introduced a difficult component in your life, it is important for you to build on those things which were important to you before. There will be a period of time, and perhaps especially in the period after being diagnosed, when it may be difficult to re-orientate yourself to the new circumstances. It may be helpful to talk through positive ways forward with someone close to you, or perhaps with a counsellor, or others with MS who may be going through the same process as yourself.

Many people find that having MS can actually create opportunities as they meet people and get involved in things which they would not have done otherwise. This can be a rich source of social contact and friendships.

If you present yourself as a person with a rich range of ideas, attitudes and opinions, you will soon find like-minded people with whom you can make friends.

Should I tell other people I meet about my diagnosis?
My symptoms are not yet very obvious to people who don't know me, but I always feel that I have to tell others at some time.

This is something which each individual has to decide for themselves depending on their particular circumstances. In general, it is better to be open about your diagnosis – particularly with close friends and family; but you should not feel obliged to tell everyone you meet by any means. It is probably best to talk to those people closest to you initially, and to tell others just as you wish or as the opportunity arises – although if you make a special point of telling people when you first meet them, and appear very awkward or very earnest about your MS, then you are likely to get a different response than if you appear to be treating MS as just a part of your life.

Be prepared to answer questions about what MS is and how it affects you. People's initial reactions may, of course, mask their own concern about how to respond as much as anything else as people often find it very difficult to know what to say. Having a few stock phrases and replies of your own to ease the situation can be a big help.

I had a very busy social life before I was diagnosed with MS.
Now I am trying to keep everything going, and I'm finding it
very difficult. Am I going to lose my friends?

Given the pressures of various combinations of social, family and work commitments, many people find that there is not only not enough time in the day to do everything, but fatigue – or other symptoms – set in and further limit what they can really do. Although it may not seem like it, if you think seriously about the balance of the things you do, you will probably find that you can prioritise your various activities.

You might also need to plan some periods of time when you can relax and rest, which may initially be frustrating for you, but is necessary to maintain your other commitments. Social events can then be made more special, and your friends will appreciate the fact that you have made them a priority.

RELATIONSHIPS WITH HEALTHCARE PROFESSIONALS

In the course of MS and its treatment, people with MS – and their relatives – often have questions and concerns about their relationship with their medical and healthcare practitioners. In this section, we address some of these worries.

Now I know that I have MS, who is really responsible for looking after me?

Once you have been diagnosed with MS (usually by a neurologist) you will usually remain under their care; this does not mean that you always see the neurologist – often they will work alongside an MS nurse and it is often the MS nurse who will be your first point of contact if you have any problems. The MS nurse can give you advice, support and information and can refer you onto other health and social care professionals as you need them (e.g. the physio, speech therapist, continence nurse and even the neurologist).

Your GP will also remain an important person in managing your care and while their knowledge of MS may not be extensive (they cannot know everything about everything after all) they will be able to liaise with your neurologist and MS nurse and help you access the care you need when you need it.

It is also important that you take responsibility for managing your

Multidisciplinary Management of Multiple Sclerosis

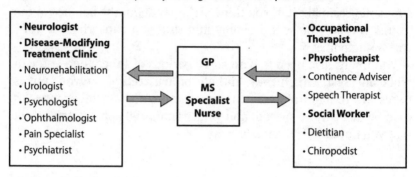

Figure 22.1 The different professionals involved in managing your MS

MS yourself – this does not mean that you should cope on your own but rather that you need to let someone know if you are having problems and need help with any aspect of your MS. Your MS nurse can usually help you with this.

I don't feel I am getting along very well with my GP. I don't think she understands me or my MS. Can I change to another GP?

In theory you can change your GP at any time simply by registering with another GP. Obviously if you cannot form an effective working relationship with your GP, then this is a good last resort, but building a rapport with any doctor may take a great deal of time and effort by both parties. MS is not an easy condition to manage, because it throws up many symptoms over its course that can need considerable medical attention or advice. Thus, for a hard-pressed GP, you may be considered to be rather a complex patient. While this should not put you off consulting your GP about symptoms that worry you, it may be sensible to consider other sources of medical advice and support where possible. An MS nurse is a good alternative in helping you to manage your MS and its impact – your MS nurse can also liaise with your GP, providing expert advice and keeping her informed about your care.

If you still wish to change your GP, then in practice this depends on whether you can find another GP who is willing to take you. In most areas of the UK, this is unlikely to be a problem, although it may involve some time on the telephone, and you do need to bear in mind that a potential GP will have to take into account that you may be a heavy user of his or her time and the practice services. However, if there is any difficulty in changing your GP, you should consult your local Primary Care Trust (or Health Board in Scotland and Wales) which oversees the operation of health services in each area.

Can I ask for a second opinion without upsetting my doctor?

Second opinions are an important part of all clinical practice, and doctors will review cases with their colleagues as a matter of course. If you wish to seek a second opinion, then you can do so through your GP, who should provide a referral and possibly make the appointment on your behalf. It is not likely that simply asking for a second opinion will upset any doctor.

What tips would you give me for getting the most out of my visit to my doctor?

You are quite likely to have only one or two appointments each year with the neurologist (at most – many people with MS just see the MS nurse and then see the neurologist if they have a particular problem which the neurologist can help with). It is important, therefore, that you are able to make the most of the appointment time.

It might be helpful to jot down beforehand the problems you are having and the issues you would like to discuss with your doctor. Remember that if you go in with a long list of problems you are unlikely to get the time to go through everything, so you should put them in order of priority. It may also be useful to discuss your list with your partner before your appointment as sometimes others see concerns which you haven't included.

When you have your appointment, do ask the doctor to explain anything that they discuss which you don't understand. Doctors are generally very good nowadays at explaining to you all the different treatment options available to help you and at discussing potential side effects of any treatments with you. It is a big help for the doctor if you can provide a list of any medications you are currently taking and the dosage, as well as approximate dates of any relapses over the last couple of years.

The doctor may well be able to provide you with a patient information leaflet covering any treatments he or she recommends, although these are not always available. It is often a good idea to make a note of what you have discussed as soon as you can after your appointment. Many doctors are now happy to send you copies of any letters arising from your appointment, so do ask about this if you would like to receive these.

There is now a wealth of information available on the Internet and there is little more likely to make a doctor's heart sink than someone coming in for their appointment clutching a thick handful of printouts from their computer. By all means discuss information you have found on the Internet if you wish but be realistic about what your doctor can read and advise you on during an appointment. Don't forget that your MS nurse can often get back to you with advice about information found on the Internet if given the opportunity to read and research the subject a little first.

If you have particular concerns, or have had an appointment with your doctor and are not sure what has been said or did not get the opportunity to discuss everything you wanted to, it is worth contacting your MS nurse who can usually help with this.

When I was having diagnostic tests for MS, and when I had a subsequent attack, my neurologist admitted me to hospital for a few days; yet my friend with MS – who has a different neurologist – has hardly spent any time in hospital at all. Why is that?

Different neurologists will work in different ways and some will tend to arrange admission to hospital more often than others. Whether you are admitted to hospital will also depend on local resources, on the exact nature and severity of your problems, and on your personal circumstances. Sometimes it can speed up access to investigations such as MRI scanning if you are admitted as an in-patient. Your neurologist may also wish to admit you for treatment with high dose steroids if you are having a relapse, although again this can often be managed either with tablets you can take at home or as a day case.

Most of the care and treatment of people with MS is now delivered either via out-patients or in the home, with in-patient admissions being kept to a minimum; however if you have any queries about where your care is being given, then do discuss this with either your neurologist or the MS nurse.

Glossary

This glossary provides brief explanations of the various technical words used in this book. Words printed in *italic* type have their own glossary entry.

action tremor An involuntary trembling or shaking of a muscle or muscle group which is more noticeable during movement than when the muscle is at rest. Some degree of *tremor* is normal for all people, but a tremor that interferes with ordinary activity may be a symptom of a neurological condition.

activities of daily living (ADLs) A set of activities essential to independent living, such as washing, dressing and eating. Some particular sets of activities and procedures for measuring the performance of them have become established as assessments of the degree of disability caused by MS. ADL scores may be used to record the progress of MS, to assess domestic needs or to test the effects of drugs in clinical trials.

acute disseminated encephalomyelitis (ADEM) An illness of the central nervous system in which one big episode of inflammation occurs, often following a viral infection. An episode of ADEM can occasionally be followed by later development of MS, but more usually ADEM is a one-off illness. ADEM is more common in children than in adults.

alemtuzumab Also known as Campath or Mab-Campath, this is a monoclonal antibody drug that has been shown to reduce MS relapses and reduce the number of new changes seen on MRI scans. Alemtuzumab is more effective, at least in the short term, than *beta-interferon* but carries greater risks. Treatment trials of alemtuzumab that are in progress should give more information about its safety.

allodynia Hot or cold sensations feeling abnormally painful.

amantadine A tablet that has been shown sometimes to improve fatigue in people with MS.

ambulant Able to walk unassisted, with or without a walking aid (a stick or frame, for instance).

anaemia A condition in which the blood does not contain enough red blood cells or enough of the pigment, haemoglobin, that carries oxygen.

ankylosing spondylitis An *autoimmune condition* that mainly affects the spine.

antibodies Substances released by a type of white blood cell called the *B-lymphocyte*. Antibodies stick to targets on the surfaces of bacteria as part of the immune system's response to fight infections. In *autoimmune conditions* like MS, antibodies may stick to the person's own cells and cause damage.

anticholinergic drugs These drugs are used in the management of urinary problems due to neurological impairment. The name refers to the way in which the drugs work – by affecting a chemical transmitter called acetylcholine, reducing spasms (contractions) in the bladder and therefore the likelihood of involuntary or too frequent urination.

antigen A part of the surface structure of biological material that can be recognised by white blood cells and to which *antibodies* may stick. Usually the antigens on the surface of cells in our bodies are recognised by our own immune system as being 'self'. The immune system is programmed not to attack 'self' antigens. In *autoimmune conditions*, including MS, this programming goes wrong, so that antibodies are made against 'self' antigens on nerves and other cells, leading to damage. White blood cells also cause damage in other ways to 'self' cells in autoimmune conditions.

auditory evoked response An electrical signal in the brain that occurs in response to sound. Tests can reveal changes in the speed, shape and distribution of these signals which are indicative of a diagnosis of MS.

autoimmune condition A disorder of the immune system in which the processes that usually defend against disease attack the body's own tissues (such as *myelin*, in the case of MS). Other autoimmune conditions include rheumatoid arthritis and *systemic lupus erythematosus* (SLE).

autologous Coming from the same organism (person) rather than from a donor.

azathioprine An old drug (given as a tablet) that has been shown to have some effectiveness as a treatment for MS, probably mainly or wholly by reducing relapses. Azathioprine has never been directly compared with *beta-interferon*, but the risks of its long-term use are probably greater than for beta-interferon.

benign MS MS which is either mild (possibly displaying no active symptoms) or in which there is little or no evidence of progressively more severe symptoms, decades after the person is diagnosed with MS. 'Benign' MS is therefore a diagnosis that can only be made in retrospect.

beta-blockers A class of drugs (known more fully as beta-adrenergic blocking agents) commonly used to treat high blood pressure, irregular heart beat and angina. Beta-blockers are sometimes used to treat *tremor* in conditions such as MS.

beta-interferon Also known as interferon beta, this is a drug that has been shown to reduce MS relapse rate by about one third. There are three main brands – Avonex, *Rebif* and Betaferon. Beta-interferon is a naturally occurring substance that is involved in the body's response to infection.

bipolar affective disorder Known previously as manic-depressive disorder, a condition that is characterised by extreme and unpredictable mood swings.

blood-brain barrier (BBB) The barrier separating the brain from the blood supplying it. In normal circumstances, essential nutrients can cross the barrier from the blood into the brain and waste products cross from the brain into the blood, but the cells of the brain are shielded from potentially harmful substances in the blood itself.

B-lymphocyte (or B-cell) A form of white blood cell that makes antibodies.

bowel incontinence see *faecal incontinence*.

brainstem The part of the brain that lies at the top of the spinal cord, connecting the spinal cord to the main substance of the brain. Damage to the brainstem may cause a number of symptoms including; *vertigo*, unsteadiness, double vision, facial weakness and numbness or speech difficulties.

cannabinoids Chemicals derived from *cannabis* plants or chemically related to them. Types of cannabinoids can be found naturally within the body, and synthetic man-made cannabinoids such as *nabilone* (*Cesamet*) are now available.

cannabis A plant species which contains many substances called *cannabinoids*, which possess a number of properties, including pain-relief, modulation of blood pressure and pulse, increased appetite and a euphoric effect which leads some people to use cannabis as a recreational drug. The use of cannabis is illegal in the UK and cannabis has been rescheduled as a Class B drug. This means the maximum penalty for possession is five years in prison and an unlimited fine.

cannabis-based medicines Pharmaceutical standard products containing specified amounts of a *cannabinoid* or cannabinoids, whether derived from cloned *cannabis* plants or man made (synthetic).

carbamazepine Also known as Tegretol, this is an anti-epileptic drug that may be used to treat pain in neurological conditions such as MS.

cardiovascular Relating to the heart and blood vessels.

CBD/cannabidiol A *cannabinoid* which reduces some side effects of tetrahydrocannabinol (THC) as well as having properties, including pain-relieving effects, of its own.

central nervous system The brain, *optic nerves* and spinal cord – these are the areas that may be affected by MS. The nerves in our arms and legs are part of the *peripheral nervous system* and are not directly affected by MS.

cerebellum A part of the brain that is involved in coordination and balance. The cerebellum lies at the base of the brain behind the *brainstem*.

cerebrospinal fluid (CSF) The fluid that surrounds the spinal column and circulates through the brain via spaces called ventricles. The CSF contains proteins, cells and chemicals that can aid the diagnosis of neurological disorders and differentiate MS from other conditions with similar or overlapping symptoms. A sample of CSF can be taken in a test called a *lumbar puncture*.

chi (qi) In Chinese medicine, the essential life-force or energy flowing in the body, imbalance of which is said to result in the symptoms of disease or illness.

chronic Long-standing or long-lasting.

clinical trial A scientific study that usually involves the testing of a drug or some other treatment in a group of people who have a medical condition.

clonazepam A drug similar to valium that is occasionally used to treat *tremor*, *spasticity* or *trigeminal neuralgia*.

clinical Relating to the examination, assessment or treatment of patients. A clinical effect is one that can be detected by the patient as a change in symptoms, or by the doctor or nurse when they examine the patient. In contrast, some treatments may affect the results of scans or blood tests without causing a clinical change.

clinically isolated syndrome (CIS) This is the first attack of inflammation in someone who may then go on to have further problems and therefore be diagnosed with MS. A CIS usually affects the *optic* (eye) nerve, the *brainstem* or *cerebellum*, or the spinal cord. Some people will only have this one episode and will not develop MS – it will remain a clinically isolated syndrome.

cognitive Relating to such things as memory, information processing, planning and problem solving These mental abilities can be affected in some people with MS.

cognitive behavioural therapy A form of psychotherapy in which the patient and therapist work in a way that is designed to change the interplay of thoughts, behaviour and emotions, so as to lead to an improvement in symptoms or a better ability to cope with these symptoms.

computerised axial tomography (CAT or CT) scan A form of detailed X-ray imaging involving radiation and multiple exposures at different positions and angles throughout the same part of the body. Computerised manipulation of the exposures results in images of structures such as the skull and brain. *MRI scanning* has replaced CT scanning as the investigation of choice when looking for conditions like MS.

contracture Shortening or shrinkage of tissue (such as connective or muscular tissue) which may result from inflammation caused by MS and which can restrict movement of joints. Exercises to maintain the flexibility of joints are particularly important because contractures may be made worse by lack of joint use.

copaxone Also known as glatiramer or glatiramer acetate, this is a *disease-modifying drug* that has been shown to reduce *relapse* rate in *relapsing-remitting MS* by about one third. The drug is given as a daily *subcutaneous* injection.

corpus callosum The central part of the brain that contains nerve fibres connecting the left side of the brain with the right side. Abnormalities in the corpus callosum on *MRI scans* are often seen in people with MS.

corticosteroids A naturally occurring group of hormones made by the adrenal gland. Large doses of corticosteroids (or 'steroids') – usually in the form of a drip or tablets of *methylprednisolone* – have been shown to speed recovery from an MS *relapse*.

CUPID A clinical trial in the UK which is testing the possibility that *cannabis*-based medicines may slow the progression of *secondary* and *primary progressive MS*.

cyclophosphamide A strong and quite dangerous *immunosuppressive drug* that is occasionally used in very aggressive cases of MS to try to achieve stabilisation of the condition.

demyelination The process of damage to the protective sheath surrounding nerves, damage to or loss of which leads to many of the symptoms of MS. The breakdown of *myelin* leads to poor or weak messages to various parts of the body and may result, in the case of MS, to the formation of plaques in which there is hardened – *sclerotic* – nerve tissue.

Devic's disease An inflammatory disorder which usually affects the spinal cord and optical (eye) nerves. It is sometimes confused with MS.

dexamethasone A form of steroid occasionally used in the treatment of MS relapses.

Disability Living Allowance (DLA) A benefit that people may be able to claim if they have walking difficulty or need help to care for themselves.

disease-modifying drug (DMD) Also known as disease-modifying treatment (DMT). These terms refer to drugs like *beta-interferon, glatiramer acetate* and *natalizumab*, which alter –'modify'– the course of MS by reducing *relapse* rate, and possibly delaying the onset of progressive problems.

double-blinded In a double-blinded drug trial, neither the patient nor the assessing doctor or nurse knows which treatment (e.g. placebo or active drug) the patient is receiving. Unblinding may occur if the patient or assessor correctly guesses what is being used. Unblinding often happens if a treatment has very obvious side effects.

EDSS (The Expanded Disability Status Scale) This is a scale used to measure disability in people with MS. It is used in most treatment trials to assess response to treatment, and is sometimes done to monitor patients in other settings.

endothelium The layer of cells that lines a hollow structure such as a blood vessel.

enhance/enhancing lesion Enhancement means that a part of the brain or spinal cord shows up more brightly on an MRI scan when *gadolinium* dye is injected into the bloodstream. The enhancement means that the dye has crossed the *blood-brain barrier*. This occurs because the inflammation in this part of the nervous system is associated with leakiness of the blood-brain barrier.

epidemiology The study of patterns of birth, death and disease within and between human populations. Often epidemiological studies try to find relationships between the frequency of MS and variations in other factors (such as diet or exposure to infections).

epidural anaesthetic Injection of anaesthetic into a space around the spinal cord. Epidural anaesthesia does not itself put someone to sleep and is sometimes used to control post-operative pain or at the time of a caesarean section.

Epstein Barr virus The virus that causes glandular fever. This virus has been linked with MS.

essential fatty acids Chemicals that are crucial for nervous system development and health. They cannot be synthesised by the body and must be obtained from the diet. Prominent essential fatty acids include linoleic, linolenic and arachidonic acids. Linolenic acid is an omega-3 fatty acid. *Linoleic acid* and arachidonic acid are omega-6 fatty acids. Essential fatty acids are found in plants and fish oils, among other sources.

Extavia A branded version of *beta-interferon* 1b, which is identical to the drug Betaferon. They differ only in their injection apparatus and support services.

faecal (bowel) incontinence The involuntary release of faeces from the bowel, resulting from constipation and partial obstruction of the bowel or from diminished control of the anal sphincter. Treatment of faecal incontinence with a bowel regimen is often successful in preventing involuntary bowel movements.

folic acid One of the B-group vitamins.

frequency The desire or need to empty the bladder often.

gabapentin An anti-epileptic drug that can be used to treat *spasticity*, pain and perhaps *tremor*.

gadolinium A contrast agent – or dye – that is sometimes injected while a patient is having an *MRI* scan. If inflammation has caused opening of the *blood-brain barrier*, the gadolinium crosses from the blood into this area of the central nervous system. This causes the corresponding area of the scan to light up, or '*enhance*'. Enhancement usually only happens in a lesion that has developed in the last 1–4 weeks, where inflammation may still be very active. Enhancing lesions are sometimes referred to as 'Gad enhancing'.

glatiramer/glatiramer acetate see *copaxone*.

glial Relating to glia, which are supporting cells within the nervous system. Although they do not carry the electrical impulses themselves, glial cells are important because they nourish and support the nerve cells. Oligodendrocytes are glial cells that produce myelin. If they are damaged, then myelin starts to deteriorate. Other examples of glial cells are astrocytes (also known as astroglia) which have a structural supportive role and also can cause scarring if they are over active – and ependymal cells, which line the fluid-filled ventricles within the brain. Microglia are similar to a sort of white blood cell called a macrophage, but live in the central nervous system rather than in the blood system. Microglia are involved in the inflammatory damage that occurs in MS relapses and in the more gradual progression of disability that sometimes occurs.

grey matter The parts of the brain and spinal cord that contain large numbers of nerve cell bodies. The cerebral cortex (the thinking part of the brain, that lies on the surface) and collections of nuclei like the thalamus which is deep within the brain are examples of grey matter structures.

herpes simplex The virus that causes cold sores and genital herpes.

hesitancy An involuntary delay or inability to start urinating.

HRT Hormone replacement therapy. Female hormones (such as oestrogens and progestogens) which can be used to treat menopausal and post-menopausal problems.

Hughes' syndrome Also known as antiphospholipid syndrome or APL, this is an autoimmune condition in which the blood has an increased tendency to clot. As a result, affected individuals have an increased risk of unusual forms of stroke. It is sometimes associated with *lupus* (*SLE*). The MRI features of Hughes' syndrome are occasionally confused with those of MS.

immunosuppressive drugs Drugs which suppress the body's natural immune responses. They have been widely used in MS in an attempt to control the damaging effects of the immune system in this *autoimmune* condition.

improved case ascertainment Sometimes people may have MS, but have never been diagnosed. Improved case ascertainment is the increased ability of the medical services to identify correctly such existing cases which have been previously undetected.

incidence of disease The measure of how often new cases of a disease are diagnosed within a population over a given time period. Incidence is usually reported per 100,000 people per year.

incontinence Loss of control of bladder or bowel function. Incontinence may result in occasional accidents or in more serious loss of voluntary control of urination or bowel movements.

inflammation Activity of the immune system, involving antibody production and the gathering of large numbers of white blood cells in tissue. As a result of the actions of the antibodies, the white cells and the chemicals they release, the area affected by inflammation will often be damaged. In the nervous system this means demyelination, axonal damage and the formation of scars by *glial* cells. Sometimes inflammation may be beneficial, by removing debris and allowing tissue repair to proceed more quickly.

inflammatory bowel disease This term refers to ulcerative colitis and Crohn's disease, conditions in which there is inflammation in the bowel wall.

interferon-beta see *beta-interferon*.

intramuscular injections Injections given within or into a muscle as opposed to intravenously (directly into a vein). Avonex, a brand of beta-interferon is given once weekly as an intramuscular injection.

isoniazid A drug used to treat tuberculosis that has been reported to help tremor in MS, but is rarely used for this purpose.

labile Volatile or unstable. 'Emotional lability', i.e. unpredictable or changeable moods, occurs in some people with MS.

latitude effect An often-repeated observation in MS research that there is a relationship between the *incidence* of MS and the distance from the equator (or latitude in geography). In other words, the further you go from the equator, the more MS cases there are. The nature of the relationship has not been fully unravelled, and there are many explanations as to why it might exist.

lesion An area of damage (in the central nervous system). This term is often used when describing MRI appearances, as it makes no assumption about the cause and nature of the damage, unlike 'plaque' which alludes to *demyelination*.

Lhermitte's phenomenon This is an electrical sensation travelling down the body when the head is bent forward. It is thought that nerves that have lost their myelin are over excitable and become activated when they are stretched as the neck is flexed. It can occur in a variety of conditions that damage the nerves at the back of the spinal cord in the neck.

licensed drugs Medicinal compounds licensed by the Committee on the Safety of Medicines for general use within medical practice in respect of particular illnesses – in other words, licensed drugs also have licensed purposes. Not all legally available drugs are licensed, such as new, untested drugs and some private treatments, supplements and complementary treatments.

linoleic acid An omega-6 essential fatty acid. Linoleic acid can be bought in chemists and health food shops, and is sometimes used as a dietary supplement.

lumbar puncture (spinal tap) A procedure in which a hollow needle is inserted into the spinal canal between two vertebrae in the lower back, in order to withdraw a sample of *cerebrospinal fluid* for analysis.

lupus see *SLE*.

magnetic field therapy As the name suggests, this is a form of complementary medicine in which magnetic fields are used in an attempt to treat an illness.

magnetic resonance imaging (MRI) A procedure in which a magnetic field, generated inside a large cylinder in which the person to be examined lies, produces detailed images of fine structures within the body. Unlike X-ray imaging, MRI can image soft tissue such as the brain, spinal column and blood vessels and does not involve exposure to radiation.

meridians Lines of energy running through the body, connecting the different anatomical sites, upon which much traditional Chinese medicine is based.

methylprednisolone A form of *steroid* that is often used to treat MS *relapses*.

metabolic Related to the biochemical processes of the body.

micturition Another word for urination.

mitoxantrone Also known as Novantrone, this strong *immunosuppressive* drug has been shown to be effective at reducing inflammation and relapses in very active cases of MS. There are significant risks in using mitoxantrone, including heart damage and a 1:300 to 1:350 risk of leukaemia. This means treatment can only be given for a short period of time, typically 3–12 months.

monoclonal antibody A pure form of antibody, usually manufactured artificially. Examples include currently available drugs like *natalizumab* and drugs in development such as *alemtuzumab*, rituximab and daclizumab, which are monoclonal antibodies targeted against different cells of the immune system.

MS nurse A nurse with special training and expertise related to MS (also referred to as MSSN or multiple sclerosis specialist nurse).

multidisciplinary team A group of professionals that may include nurses, doctors (of various specialties), *occupational therapists*, physiotherapists, speech and language therapists, social workers and psychologists.

multimodal therapy A form of behavioural and psychological intervention pioneered by South African psychologist Arnold Lazarus in which seven different aspects (modalities) of personality and psychology may be addressed. The seven modalities are: Behaviour, Affect (mood), Sensation, Imagery, Cognition (thinking and reasoning), Interpersonal relationships, and Drugs/biology.

myasthenia gravis An autoimmune condition that affects eye muscles, limb muscles, speech, swallowing and sometimes breathing.

myelin A fatty layer that forms the outer part of many of the larger nerves in the human body. Myelin acts as an electrical insulator, thereby enabling nerves coated by it to carry electrical impulses more quickly and efficiently. See also *demyelination*.

myelitis Inflammation of the spinal cord. Partial myelitis affects the spinal cord in only part of its cross-sectional area, giving rise to asymmetric symptoms. Transverse myelitis affects the whole cross-section of the spinal cord and causes more severe and symmetrical problems below that level, by preventing normal electrical transmission through this inflamed section of the spinal cord.

nabilone (Cesamet) Synthetic tetrahydrocannabinol (THC), a *cannabinoid*, licensed in the UK for nausea and vomiting in people receiving chemotherapy.

natalizumab A disease-modifying drug for actively relapsing MS which reduces the relapse rate by about two-thirds. Natalizumab is a *monoclonal antibody* that reduces the ability of white blood cells to bind to and cross the blood-brain barrier, thereby reducing the number of MS relapses. The trade name for this drug is Tysabri.

neuralgia Abnormal, dagger-like pains caused by damage to, or disturbance in function of, a nerve.

neural therapy A form of complementary medicine that has some similarities to acupuncture. In neural therapy, parts of the body may be injected with local anaesthetics or homeopathic substances.

neurofibromatosis A rare condition in which there are multiple benign tumours that develop from nerves.

neurological examination An evaluation of the function of the nervous system. A neurological assessment is essential to the diagnosis of MS and will (at least initially) involve the elimination of other conditions with similar symptoms. The assessment will include the taking of a medical history and examination of reflexes, senses and functional abilities.

neuromyelitis optica See *Devic's disease.*

neuron A nerve cell.

neuropathic pain Pain that is due to some kind of damage to, or disease in, the nerves that sense pain. Neuropathic pain will often happen in the absence of stimuli or be induced by stimuli that are not normally painful. It is also often different in character from other types of pain.

neutralising antibodies (NABs) These are antibodies made by the body which have the effect of blocking the benefits of a treatment. They can be present and raise management issues for people who are on *beta-interferon* or, less commonly, for people on *natalizumab.*

NICE (National Institute for Health and Clinical Excellence) An independent body established by the British Government to assess the effectiveness of healthcare interventions in relation to their cost. The intention is that only interventions (including drugs) approved by NICE will be available through the NHS.

nystagmus An involuntary, jerking movement of the eyes resulting (in the case of MS) from damage to the nervous system. Nystagmus can result in severe visual problems that make reading extremely tiring or difficult.

occupational therapist (OT) A health care professional who has expertise in helping people adapt themselves and their environment in order to cope better with problems arising from their medical condition. Occupational therapists also have a role in devising activities that help people to recover better from an episode of illness.

oligoclonal bands (OCBs) *Antibodies* found in the spinal fluid of more than 90 per cent of people with MS. They are also seen in some other inflammatory neurological conditions.

ondansetron A strong anti-nausea drug that has occasionally been used to treat *tremor*.

optic neuritis Inflammation of the optic nerve (behind the eye). Optic neuritis can result in reduced or blurred vision, impaired colour perception as well as pain and tenderness.

osteoporosis Thinning of the bones which makes them more vulnerable to breaking. People with MS are at increased risk of osteoporosis if they are regularly treated with *steroids*, or if they are unable to exercise regularly.

palliative care The branch of health care that is concerned with alleviating symptoms, especially in those who are very unwell or disabled.

PASAT The Paced Auditory Serial Addition Test – a test that is sometimes used in clinical trials. The PASAT gives information about how quickly people can process information with their brain.

Phase 1, Phase 2 and Phase 3 clinical trials Phase 1 trials are often conducted on small numbers of healthy volunteers, to get an early idea as to the safety of a drug. Phase 2 studies are the first assessment as to whether a drug may work, but are not usually big enough or long enough to prove that a drug has major benefits. Phase 3 studies are large scale trials performed using drugs that have shown promise in Phases 1 and 2 trials, to try and prove whether they really are beneficial.

placebo A biologically inactive substance used as a dummy drug (or 'control') in a clinical trial. Placebos can have real effects on people, presumably because they make people feel optimistic that there may be an improvement in their condition.

plaque An area of the central nervous system that has been damaged by inflammatory MS activity. The plaque is characterised by loss *of myelin*, variable loss of *axons*, and *glial* scarring and will sometimes show up as a white dot on an *MRI* scan.

prednisolone A form of *steroid*, usually given in tablet form and occasionally used in the treatment of MS *relapses*.

pressure sores Areas of damaged skin that may be ulcerated or infected. As the name implies, pressure sores are in areas that a patient sits or lies on, like the heels or the buttocks. Pressure sores typically develop in people who are less able to move around or turn over.

prevalence A measure of the proportion of the population with a given condition, often expressed as the number of cases of the condition for each thousand people of the population. This measure allows comparison of the frequency of the condition between populations of different sizes.

primary progressive MS A type of MS characterised by a pattern of progressively more severe or widespread symptoms over time, without *relapses*.

primidone An old anti-epileptic drug that is still occasionally used to treat *tremor*.

prognosis An educated assessment of the likely future course of a medical condition and its effects. No prognosis can ever be more than a good guess based on prior experience, and may include both best and worst case outcomes.

progressive multi-focal leukoencephalopathy (PML) A life-threatening brain viral infection affecting people who have an underactive immune system, including those on immunosuppressive medication.

pseudo-relapse a worsening of symptoms in MS that is due to something other than a new episode of inflammation. Pseudo-relapses usually have no completely new features and are particularly likely to happen when a person with MS has an infection.

psoriasis An *autoimmune condition* in which there are skin and sometimes joint problems.

pulmonary embolism A blood clot in an artery in the lungs.

qi see *chi*.

randomisation A process in which patients enrolled into a drug trial are allocated without any bias to the different arms (for example, *placebo* versus active treatment) of the trial.

Rebif One of the makes of *beta-interferon*, Rebif is a subcutaneous injection of beta-interferon 1A, given three times a week.

reflexology A form of complementary therapy in which manipulation of the feet is designed to improve the symptoms or progression of a medical condition.

relapse An episode of inflammation that results in a new problem or problems for an individual with MS.

relapsing-remitting MS A type of MS which is characterised by *relapses*, followed by *remissions* in which there is a partial or full recovery from these symptoms. In some cases complete recovery may occur from all symptoms, but in other cases recovery is partial. Relapses may occur every few months or may be years apart.

remission The period of time between *relapses* when no new symptoms are developing.

remyelination Restoration, or partial restoration, of the insulating *myelin* sheath around a nerve axon, allowing the axon to conduct electricity more effectively. The human central nervous system has some capacity to remyelinate demyelinated nerves, but full remyelination is unusual.

respite care The opportunity for a patient to attend a nursing home or some other kind of supervised facility. This may mean that the patient's main carer(s) can do things that would not be possible if the respite care were not available.

rheumatoid arthritis An *autoimmune condition* in which joints are affected.

rituximab A *monoclonal antibody* that sticks to *B-lymphocytes* and consequently reduces the number of them. Rituximab has shown promise in a preliminary trial in *relapsing-remitting MS*.

risk sharing scheme The Department of Health Risk Sharing scheme was set up in 2002 so that *beta-interferon* (Avonex, Betaferon and *Rebif*) and *glatiramer acetate (Copaxone)* would be funded by local health authorities for use in MS patients who might benefit. In the scheme, patients started on treatment between 2002 and 2005 will have annual assessments when the number of relapses and the degree of disability will be recorded. The scheme is intended to run for at least 10 years, and patients will still be monitored in the scheme even if they stop or switch disease-modifying treatment.

rubella German measles.

sarcoidosis A rare condition in which inflammation may develop in various tissues, including the skin, lungs and central nervous system. Occasionally, sarcoidosis can be mistaken for MS, and *vice versa*.

sativex A *cannabis*-based medicine made from cannabis plants with genetically determined amounts of tetrahydrocannabinol (THC) and cannabidiol (CBD) mixed in roughly 1:1 proportions, dissolved into liquid form and taken as a spray applied to the inside of the cheek.

secondary progressive MS A type of MS in which, following initially *benign* or *relapsing-remitting MS*, symptoms then begin to progress steadily.

sensory symptoms Symptoms which involve a problem with one of the senses – touch, taste, smell, hearing and sight. All senses may be affected in MS, although visual symptoms and disturbances of touch and pain perception are more frequently reported than problems with hearing, taste or smell and are most likely to impact on activities of daily living.

shiatzu A form of massage based on the pressure treatment (acupressure) of the same points used in acupuncture treatment.

SNRIs Abbreviation for selective noradrenaline reuptake inhibitors – a type of antidepressant drug that can also be used to treat some types of neuropathic (nerve) pain.

SP Short for *secondary progressive*.

spasticity Stiffness or tension in muscles that is not caused by excessive exercise, and in MS is usually caused by the continuing effects of abnormal nervous system control of the relevant muscles.

specific A medical test that is 100 per cent specific for a condition will only be positive in people who have that condition. In reality, even a good test is usually only 90 per cent specific. In contrast, the term 'sensitive' refers to the percentage of patients with a certain condition that will be picked up by a test. A test which is 80 per cent sensitive would be positive in 8 out of 10 individuals with the condition, but could still be 100 per cent specific if it never gave a positive result in someone without the condition.

spina bifida A developmental disorder or 'birth defect' in which the spinal column has not developed normally.

spinal cord The spinal cord is a large collection of nerves running in the back – in the spinal canal – from the neck down to the lower back. Damage to the spinal cord in the neck – for example, due to inflammation in someone with MS – may cause weakness, numbness and lost or altered feeling in the arms and legs. Spinal cord problems need not be symmetrical. Indeed, in a typical episode of partial *myelitis* due to MS, the symptoms are often worse on one side than the other.

steroids See *corticosteroids*.

subcutaneously Under the skin. A subcutaneous injection is given in the tissues immediately beneath the skin. Betaferon and *Rebif*, two brands of *beta-interferon*, are given either on alternate days or three times weekly, respectively, as subcutaneous injections.

systemic lupus erythematosus (SLE) An *autoimmune condition* that affects joints, skin, kidneys and sometimes the nervous system.

T'ai chi A Chinese process that combines physical exercises similar to Yoga, with meditation.

THC tetrahydrocannabinol One of the active chemicals produced by the *cannabis* plant, thought to be the main cause of the effects sought by recreational users of cannabis.

tissue viability nurse A nurse with special training to help people with mobility problems reduce their risk of developing *pressure sores* and to help people recover from pressure sores.

titration Adjusting medication cautiously, usually by increasing the dose, to find the dose which gives the best balance between good effects and side effects.

T-lymphocytes (or T-cells) White blood cells that can directly attack bacteria, helping fight off infections. In MS, T-cells cross the *blood-brain barrier*, entering the *central nervous system* where they are involved in the inflammation that causes damage to nerves.

topiramate Also known as Topamax. An anti-epileptic drug that can also be used to prevent migraine and may have a role in the treatment of *tremor* in MS.

tremor An involuntary shaking or trembling of muscles at rest or (more commonly in MS) during movement.

tricyclic antidepressant drugs Drugs like *amitriptyline* that are sometimes used to treat pain in people with neurological conditions like MS.

trigeminal neuralgia This is pain associated with abnormal activity of the trigeminal nerve – the nerve supplying the cheek, lips, gums and chin. The pain is usually intense, stabbing, brief and associated with only one side of the face.

Tysabri See *natalizumab*.

urgency The desire or need to pass urine immediately. Urgency is not necessarily associated with a full bladder, but is nevertheless almost impossible to ignore.

Uhthoff's phenomenon. A temporary disturbance of vision that may follow vigorous exercise. The same sort of effect is also observed with increases in body temperature due to any cause and can affect any set of symptoms.

vasculitis Inflammation in blood vessels. When vasculitis affects blood vessels in the brain, stroke-like episodes may happen.

VER See *visual evoked response.*

vertigo A disorientating sensation of unsteadiness. The world often appears to be spinning. It may sometimes be described as a dizzy spell. Vertigo results from a disturbance of the fluid in the inner ear or from a disorder of the nerves carrying signals from the inner ear to the brain.

vestibular system The system involved in sensing head position and controlling balance. It operates through fluid-filled canals in the inner ear and the nerve carrying signals from the inner ear to the brain.

visual evoked potential (VEP) See *visual evoked response.*

visual evoked response (VER) An electrical signal in the brain that occurs in response to an image. Recordings of responses to test patterns, often of regular patterns of black and white squares or lines of different sizes, can be used to determine the nature and location of abnormalities of visual pathways. VERs are sometimes used to help make a diagnosis of MS.

vitamin B12 A vitamin that is needed for healthy blood and nerves. Deficiency of B12, often due to an *autoimmune condition* called pernicious *anaemia*, may lead to progressive neurological problems that share some features with MS.

white matter The parts of the brain and spinal cord that contain large numbers of nerve fibres. The *myelin* on many of the nerve fibres gives this tissue a paler appearance than the *grey matter*.

| Appendix 1
Useful addresses

Multiple sclerosis

MS Society and MS Trust

The MS Society of Great Britain and Northern Ireland

The MS Society is the largest national society providing help, information, advice and funding for people living with and working with MS. It has a network of local branches across the UK which can be sourced via the Society's award winning website or helpline. Through its branches, the MS Society undertakes a great deal of welfare work locally with people living with MS. At a national level it also funds a great deal of research into cause, cure, care and symptomatic relief of MS.

The MS Society National Centre
373 Edgware Road
London NW2 6ND
Helpline: 0808 800 8000
Email: helpline@mssociety.org.uk
Website: www.mssociety.org.uk

MS Society Scotland
Ratho Park
88 Glasgow Road
Ratho Station
Newbridge
EH28 8PP
Tel: 0131 335 4050
Fax: 0131 335 4051
Website www.mssocietyscotland.org.uk

MS Society Wales/Cymru
Temple Court
Cathedral Road
Cardiff
CF11 9HA
Tel: 029 2078 6676
Fax: 029 2078 6677
Email: mscymruwales@mssociety.org.uk

MS Society Northern Ireland Office
The Resource Centre
34 Annadale Avenue
Belfast BT7 3JJ
Tel: 028 9080 2802
Website: www.mssocietyni.co.uk

The Multiple Sclerosis Trust

The MS Trust is a large national society which provides information and advice for people living with MS, and education and various resources for health professionals working with people affected by MS. The Society's website contains a wealth of resources for people affected by MS and for health professionals alike.

The MS Trust

Spirella Building
Bridge Road
Letchworth Garden City
Hertfordshire
SG6 4ET
Tel: 01462 476700
Fax: 01462 476710
Email: info@mstrust.org.uk
Website: www.mstrust.org.uk

Other MS-related organisations

British Trust for the Myelin Project

139 Hulme Hall Road
Cheadle Hulme
Stockport SK8 6LQ
Tel: 0161 292 3191
Website: www.myelinproject.co.uk
The Myelin Project is an international, non-profit partnership of neurologists, researchers and informed lay-people. The Myelin Project's purpose is to find therapies for demyelinating diseases, both acquired (such as multiple sclerosis)

and hereditary neurodegenerative disorders (the leukodystrophies). The British Trust for the Myelin Project also provides information and support to people with myelin-related conditions.

Jooly's Joint

Website: www.mswebpals.org
A forum for people of all ages who are affected by MS to talk and share information, experiences and generally chat.

MS Decisions

Website: www.msdecisions.org.uk
An independent site funded by the Department of Health containing information about the different disease-modifying therapies. It is aimed at people who have been recommended to start treatment with one of the DMTs and need more information to help them decide which of the drugs will be most appropriate for them as an individual and contains a wealth of information about these treatments.

MS First

MS Research Training
and Education Limited
10 Oakwood Road
Henleaze
Bristol BS9 4NR
Tel: 0117 342 6332
Website: www.ms-research.org.uk
A charity supporting MS research and education.

MS International Federation (MSIF)
3rd Floor, Skyline House
200 Union Street
London SE1 0LX
Tel: 020 7620 1911
Fax: 020 7620 1922
Email: info@msif.org
Website: www.misf.org
Runs a website which contains a great deal of useful information both for people affected by MS and for health professionals. There is a quarterly journal which can be downloaded or ordered free of charge covering topics such as stem cells in MS and spasticity. There is also an opportunity to subscribe to a weekly e-mail with regular updates and news from the world of MS.

The MSIF, in conjunction with the World Health Organization, has produced an Atlas of MS (Sept 2008) which is full of information about the prevalence of MS around the world and of the resources which are available in different parts of the world. This is free to download from the MSIF site or a hard copy can be purchased for a nominal sum.

MS National Therapy Centres
Website: www.ms-selfhelp.org
The MS Therapy Centres can be found across the UK and are each run at a local level. Each of the centres provides a number of different services, typically including hyperbaric oxygen tanks, physiotherapy and counselling as well as providing a focal point for people living with MS to meet each other and to source information.

Neurological Alliance
Website: www.neural.org.uk
The Neurological Alliance enables charities to work together to improve quality of life for all those living in the UK with a neurological condition. The site includes details of useful organisations, publications and information including access to the leaflet 'Getting the best from neurological services' which is published by the Alliance.

UK Multiple Sclerosis Tissue Bank
Division of Neuroscience and Mental Health
Imperial College London
Charing Cross Campus
Fulham Palace Road
London W6 8RF
Tel: 020 8846 7324
Fax: 020 8846 7500
E-mail: ukmstissuebank@imperial.ac.uk
Website: www.ukmstissuebank.org.uk
The aims of the Tissue Bank are to provide a facility for people who want to donate their organs to research, and to act as an essential resource for those scientists conducting research on the cause and treatment of multiple sclerosis.

Living with MS

Ability Net
Website: www.abilitynet.org.uk
A national charity helping disabled adults and children use computers and the internet by adapting and adjusting their technology to suit individual needs.

Association of Disabled Professionals
BCM ADP
London WC1N 3XX
Tel: 01204 431638
Fax: 01204 431638
Email: adp.admin@ntlworld.com
Promotes education, rehabilitation, training and employment opportunities available to professional people with disabilities.

Bladder & Bowel Foundation
SATRA Innovation Park
Rockingham Road
Kettering
Northants NN16 9JH
Tel: 01536 533255
Fax: 01536 533240
Nurse helpline: 0845 345 0165
Counsellor helpline: 0870 770 3246
Email: info@bladderandbowelfoundation.org
Website: bladderandbowelfoundation.org
A new charity and website designed to help people who have any problem with their bladder or bowels and for the professionals who provide services.

British Association of Counselling and Psychotherapy
BACP House
15 St John's Business Park
Lutterworth
Leicestershire LE17 4HB
Tel: 01455 883300
Fax: 01455 550243
Email: bacp@bacp.co.uk
Provides advice on a range of services to help meet the needs of anyone seeking information about counselling and psychotherapy.

Calibre Audio Library
Tel: 01296 432339
Website: www.calibre.org.uk
A free nationwide postal library of unabridged recorded books for people with sight problems or other disabilities. You do not have to be registered as having a visual impairment to be able to use this facility.

Ceiling Hoist Users Club
Website: www.chuc.org.uk
A website giving details of hoist-friendly hotels and B&Bs, and which contains a wealth of information.

Citizens Advice
Website: www.citizensadvice.org.uk
The home page for this national organisation contains large amounts of information and advice and incorporates a search facility to find details of your nearest office.

Depression Alliance
35 Westminster Bridge Road
London SE1 7JB
Tel: 020 7633 9929
Fax: 020 7633 0559
Helpline: 0845 123 2320
Website: www.depressionalliance.org.uk
Offers support and understanding to anyone affected by depression, and to relatives who want help. Has a network of self-help groups, correspondence schemes and a range of literature. Send s.a.e. for information.

Disability Alliance
First Floor East
Universal House
88–94 Wentworth Street
London E1 7SA
Tel: 020 7247 8776
Fax: 020 7247 8765
Helpline: 020 7247 8763
Website: www.disabilityalliance.org.uk
Offers a rights service on social security benefits.

Disability Equipment Register
4 Chatterterton Road
Yate
Bristol BS37 4BJ
Tel: 01454 318818
Fax: 01454 883870
Website: www.disabreg.dial.pipex.com
Nationwide service for buying and selling used disabled equipment.

Disability Sport England
Solecast House
13–27 Brunswick Place
London N1 6DX
Tel: 020 7490 4919
Fax: 020 7490 4914
Website: www.disabilitysport.org.uk

Disabled Holiday Information UK
Website: www.disabledholidayinfo.org.uk
Information about holidays for people with disabilities including wheelchair-accessible visitor attractions, activities and accommodation.

Disabled Living
Redbank House
4 St Chads Street
Cheetham
Manchester M8 8QA
Tel: 0870 7601580
Website: www.disabledliving.co.uk
Offers a comprehensive range of services to improve quality of life for disabled people including supply and advice about equipment and adaptations.

Disabled Living Foundation
380–384 Harrow Road
London W9 2HU
Helpline: 0845 130 9177 (10 am to 4 pm, Mon–Fri)
Textphone: 020 7432 8009
Email: advice@dlf.org.uk
Website: www.dlf.org.uk
Provides free, impartial advice about all types of daily living equipment and

mobility products for disabled adults and children, older people, their carers and families.

Disabled Motorists Federation
145 Knoulberry Road
Blackfell
Washington
Tyne & Wear NE37 1JN
Tel: 0191 416 3172
Fax: 0191 416 3172
Website: www.freewebs.com/dmfed
The Disabled Motorists Federation was originally formed by a number of independent small, local, disabled motorists clubs in the Midlands. The heart of the Federation consists of 12 independent clubs, plus an affiliated club based in Moscow. These are situated all over the country; they meet on a regular basis, and arrange outings for their members. They attempt to influence local councils to provide better resources for the disabled, especially in connection with motoring.

Employment Opportunities for People with Disabilities
123 Minories
London EC3N 1NT
Telephone: 020 7448 5420
Fax: 020 7374 4913
Textphone: 020 7374 6684
Email: info@eopps.org
Website: www.opportunities.org.uk
Helps people with disabilities find and retain employment through training,
mock interviews, assessment, graduate scheme and support during placements. Regional centres offer training in disability awareness to employers.

Family Fund
Unit 4, Alpha Court
Monks Cross Drive
York YO32 9WN
Tel: 0845 130 4542
Website: www.familyfund.org.uk
Helps families with severely disabled children to have choices and the opportunity to enjoy ordinary life. Gives grants for things that make life easier and more enjoyable for the disabled child and their family, such as washing machines, driving lessons, hospital visiting costs, computers and holidays.

Gardening for Disabled Trust
PO Box 285
Tunbridge Wells
Kent, TN2 9JD
Website:
www.gardeningfordisabledtrust.org.uk
Gardening can be fun again! This website is full of useful information to help people with disabilities enjoy gardening.

GLAMS
Weblink:
www.mssociety.org.uk/support_and_services/
support_groups/gay_and_lesbian.html
*A specialist group within the MS
Society (see the beginning of this
Appendix) to support gay and lesbian
people with MS.*

Mobilise
Ashwelthorpe
Norwich NR16 1EX
Tel: 01508 489 449
Fax: 01508 488 173
Website: www.dda.org.uk
*The result of a merger of the Disabled
Drivers' Association and the Disabled
Drivers' Motor Club, this organisation
provides information and advice,
aiming for independence through
mobility.*

Motability
City Gate House
22 Southwark Bridge Road
London SE1 9HB
Tel: 0845 456 4566 (8.30 am to 5.30
pm Mon – Fri)
Textphone: 0845 675 0009
Website: www.motability.co.uk
*The Motability Scheme enables
disabled people to use their
government-funded mobility
allowances to obtain a new car,
powered wheelchair or scooter and
supports adaptations of cars to meet
individual needs.*

**National Centre for Disabled
Living**
4th Floor, Hampton House
20 Albert Embankment
London SE1 7TJ
Tel: 0207 587 1663
Fax: 0207 582 2469
Text: 0207 587 1177
Email: info@ncil.org.uk
*A support, advice and consultancy
organisation (based in South London,
but working all over the country) that
aims to enable disabled people to be
equal citizens with choice, control,
rights and full economic, social and
cultural lives.*

Partially Sighted Society
PO Box 322
Doncaster DN1 2XA
Tel: 01302 323 132
Fax: 01302 368 998
*Assists visually impaired people to
make the best use of their remaining
vision with a range of useful
publications and equipment available
by mail order.*

Patients Association
PO Box 935
Harrow
Middlesex HA1 3YJ
Tel: 020 8423 9111
Tel: 020 8423 9112
Website: www.patients-association.com
Provides advice on patients' rights.

Patient UK

Website: www.patient.co.uk

Details of patient support organisations, self-help groups, health and disease information, providers, benefits and financial advice etc.

RADAR (Royal Association for Disability and Rehabilitation)

12 City Forum

250 City Road

London EC1V 8AF

Tel: 020 7250 3222

Fax: 020 7250 0212

Minicom: 020 7250 4119

Email: radar@radar.org.uk

Website: www.radar.org.uk

The UK's largest disability campaigning network, with over 900 individual and organisational members. Radar's vision is for a just and equal society whose strength is human difference. Its mission is to enable individuals, networks and policy makers to do things differently.

Relate

Herbert Gray College

Little Church Street

Rugby

Warwickshire CV21 3AP

Tel: 01788 573 241

Fax: 01788 535 007

Helpline: 0845 130 4010

Website: www.relate.org.uk

Offers relationship council via local branches. Publishes information on issues relating to health, self-esteem, sexual relationships, depression, bereavement and remarriage.

REMAP

Unit D9

Chaucer Business Park

Kemsing

Sevenoaks

Kent TN15 6YU

Tel: 0845 130 0456

Fax: 0845 130 0789

Website: www.remap.org.uk

Custom made equipment for people with a whole range of disabilities.

Riding for the Disabled (RDA)

Norfolk House

Tournament Court

Edgehill Drive

Warwick CV34 6LG

Tel: 0845 658 1082

Fax: 0845 658 1083

Website: www.riding-for-disabled.org.uk

SKILL

Tel: 0800 328 5050

Website: www.skill.org.uk

Gives information about learning, training and employment opportunities for adults and young people with any kind of disability.

Tourism for All
The Hawkins Suite
Enham Place
Enham Alamein
Andover SP11 6JS
Tel: 0845 124 9971
Fax: 0845 124 9972
Minicom: 0845 124 9976
Email: info@tourismforall.org.uk

Tripscope
The Vassall Centre
Gill Avenue
Bristol BS16 2QQ
Tel: 08457 585641
Fax: 0117 9397736
Email: tripscopesw@cableinet.co.uk
*A nationwide travel and transport
information service which helps with
information about travel, whether
planning journeys, involving private
motoring or public transport, for
people with mobility problems and
their carers.*

Vitalise
12 City Forum
250 City Road
London EC1V 8AF
Tel: 0845 345 1972
Fax: 0845 345 1978
Website: www.vitalise.org.uk
*A national charity providing short
breaks (respite care) and other
services for disabled people, visually
impaired people and carers.*

Volunteer England
Website: www.volunteering.org.uk
*Website giving information about local
and national volunteering options.*

Complementary therapies

Association of Reflexologists
5 Fore Street
Taunton
Somerset TA1 1HX
Tel: 01823 351010
Fax: 01823 336646
Email: info@aor.org.uk
Website: www.aor.org.uk
*A non-profit making membership
organisation providing support to
professionally qualified practitioners.*

British Acupuncture Council
63 Jeddo Road
London W12 9HQ
Tel: 020 8735 0400
Fax: 0 20 8735 0404
Email: info@acupuncture.org.uk
Website: www.acupuncture.org.uk
*The UK's main regulatory body for
the practice of traditional acupuncture
by over 2800 professionally qualified
acupuncturists.*

British Complementary Medicine Association
PO Box 5122
Bournemouth BH8 0WG
Tel: 0845 345 5977
Website: www.bcma.co.uk
An open-minded Association that supports any recognised therapy providing the standards of training are adequate and their codes of ethics and disciplines are adhered to. Non-profit making, reinvesting all fees for the benefit of complementary medicine and those who practise it.

British Herbal Medicine Association
PO Box 583
Exeter EX1 9GX
Tel: 0845 680 1134
Fax: 0845 680 1136
Email: secretary@bhma.info
Website: www.bhma.info
Founded in 1964 to advance the science and practice of herbal medicine in the United Kingdom and to ensure its continued statutory recognition at a time when all medicines were becoming subject to greater regulatory control.

British Holistic Medical Association
PO Box 371
Bridgwater
Somerset TA6 9BG
Tel: 01278 722 000
Email: admin@bhma.org
Website: www.bhma.org
The BHMA is an open association of mainstream healthcare professionals, CAM practitioners, and members of the public who want to adopt a more holistic approach in their own life and work.

British Homeopathic Association
Hahnemann House
29 Park Street West
Luton LU1 3BE
Tel: 0870 444 3950
Fax: 0870 444 3960
Email: info@britishhomeopathic.org
Website: www.trusthomeopathy.org
Promotes homeopathy practised by doctors and other healthcare professionals, funding their education and encouraging high quality research.

British Medical Acupuncture Association
BMAS House
3 Winnington Court
Northwich
Cheshire CW8 1AQ
Tel: 01606 786782
Fax: 01606 786783
Email: admin@medical-acupuncture.org.uk

or

Royal London Homoeopathic Hospital
60 Great Ormond St
London WC1N 3HR
Tel: 020 7713 9437
Fax: 020 7713 6286
Email: bmaslondon@aol.com
Website: www.medical-acupuncture.org.uk
Seeks to enhance the education and training of suitably qualified practitioners, and to promote high standards of working practices in acupuncture. Members are regulated healthcare professionals who practise acupuncture.

British Reflexology Association
Monks Orchard
Whitbourne
Worcester WR6 5RB
Tel: 01886 821 207
Fax: 01529 822 017
Website: www.britreflex.co.uk
Professional body offering training and list of accredited members.

British Wheel of Yoga
25 Jermyn Street
Sleaford NG34 7RU
Tel: 01529 306 851
Fax: 01529 303 233
Website: www.bwy.org.uk
Professional body offering lists of qualified yoga therapists.

General Osteopathic Council
176 Tower Bridge Road
London SE1 3LU
Tel: 020 7357 6655
Fax: 020 7357 0011
Website: www.osteopathy.org.uk
The regulatory body for osteopaths in the UK.

Institute for Complementary and Natural Medicine
Can-Mezzanine
32–36 Loman Street
London SE1 0EH
Tel: 0207 922 7980
Website: www.i-c-m.org.uk

National Institute of Medical Herbalists
Elm House
54 Mary Arches Street
Exeter EX4 3BA
Tel: 01392 426022
Fax: 01392 498963
Email: info@nimh.org.uk
Website: www.nimh.org.uk
All enquiries should be addressed to the NIMH Office at the address above.

Yoga Biomedical Trust
Fourth Floor
Royal London Homeopathic
Hospital
60 Great Ormond Street
London WC1N 3HR
Tel: 020 7149 7159

**Yoga for Healthcare
EducationTrust**
18 Haymarket
Lytham St Annes FY8 3LW
Tel: 01253 640247
Website: www.yoga-health-education.org.uk
*A charity dedicated to bringing yoga
to all. whether fit and well or disabled.*

Carers' organisations

Caring about Carers
Website: www.direct.gov.uk/en/CaringFor
Someone/index.htm
*Information provided by the
Department of Health to help and
support carers in their role.*

Carers Connect
Website: www.carersconnect.com
*A website developed for Carers and
those working in the care sector
providing access to forums, live online
chat and private messaging.*

Carers UK
20 Great Dover Street
London SE1 4LX
Tel: 020 7378 4999
Fax: 020 7378 9781
Email: info@carersuk.org
Website: www.carersuk.org
*Provides a voice for carers, and offers
information and support.*

Crossroads
Tel: 0845 450 0350
Website: www.crossroads.org.uk
*An independent charity aimed
at improving the lives of carers by
giving them time to be themselves and
have a break from their caring
responsibilities. Their aim is to provide
a reliable service, tailored to meet the
individual needs of each carer and the
person they are caring for. They have
schemes in most parts of England and
Wales which provide a range of
services to meet local needs. Local
schemes are listed in the Local
Services section.*

Crossroads in Scotland
Website: www.crossroads-scotland.co.uk
*Scotland's largest provider of short
breaks and practical support for
carers. They represent the interests of
46 local services throughout the
country that provide opportunities for
carers to take time for themselves.*

Princess Royal Trust for Carers
Websites: www.carers.org
www.youngcarers.net
The largest provider of comprehensive support services for carers in the UK. Through its unique network of 129 independently managed Carers' Centres and interactive websites, the Trust currently provides quality information, advice and support services to 290,000 carers, including just over 15,000 young carers.

Health Service and Government Departments

Department for Work and Pensions
Helpline: 0800 131 177
Government information service offering advice on benefits for people with disabilities and their carers.

Department of Health
Richmond House
79 Whitehall
London SW1A 2NS
Tel: 020 7210 4850
Website: www.dh.gov.uk

DVLA (Drivers and Vehicles Licensing Authority)
Medical Branch
Longview Road
Morriston
Swansea SA99 1TU
Tel: 0870 240 0009
Helpline: 0870 600 0301

Expert patients programme
Website: www.expertpatients.co.uk
Generic courses for people who live with long-term health conditions.

National Institute for Health and Clinical Excellence (NICE)
Website: www.nice.org.uk
The organisation responsible for providing national guidance on drugs and treatments offered in the NHS. To download or view the NICE guidelines pertinent to MS, search under 'Our Guidance' on this website.

National Service Framework
Weblink:
www.dh.gov.uk/en/Policyandguidance/Health andsocialcaretopics/Longtermconditions/Long-termNeurologicalConditionsNSF/index.htm
The NSF for Long Term Conditions which includes advice about neurological conditions can be viewed/downloaded from the Department of Health website, specifically from the link provided.

NHS Direct

Tel: 0845 4647

Website: www.nhsdirect.nhs.uk

24-hour helpline providing information and advice about health, illness and services.

Patient Advice and Liaison Service (PALS)

Website: www.pals.nhs.uk

PALS has been introduced to ensure that the NHS listens to patients, their relatives, carers and friends, and answers their questions and resolves their concerns as quickly as possible. You are advised to direct your enquiries to your local PALS, which you can find through the website above (look under 'Local PALS').

Appendix 2
Further reading and useful resources

Publications from the MS Society

MS Matters, the Society's newsletter is published monthly, and is also available on audio cassette. It is free to members. The Society also publishes many useful booklets and pamphlets, that can be ordered or downloaded free from the website. Topics covered include the following:

A guide to health care services
Adaptations and your home
Benefits and MS
Caring for someone with MS: a handbook for family and friends
Childhood MS – a guide for parents
Complementary and alternative medicine
Diet and nutrition
Disease-modifying drugs
Exercise and physiotherapy
Fatigue
Finding and funding residential care
Getting the best from social care services
Insurance and MS
Just diagnosed – an introduction to MS
Living with the effects of MS
Managing bladder and bowel problems
Managing relapses
Memory and thinking
Mood, depression and emotions
Muscle spasms and stiffness
Pain and sensory symptoms
Sex, intimacy and relationships
Speech difficulties
Support for people severely affected by MS
Swallowing difficulties

Tremor
Vision and MS
Women's health – pregnancy, menstruation, contraception and menopause
Working with MS: information for employees and employers

Publications from the MS Trust

Open Door is a free, quarterly newsletter for people with MS, their family and friends and supporters of the MS Trust. The Trust also publishes a range of free factsheets and booklets on topics such as:

Alemtuzumab (Campath)
At work with MS
Bladder problems
Bowel problems
Cannabis
Cladribine
Cognition
Conception, pregnancy and after
Diet
Disease-modifying drug therapies
Esperanza Homeopathic NeuroPeptide
Exercises for people with MS
Falls
Fatigue
Functional electrical stimulation (FES)
Getting the best from neurological services
Goat serum
Kids' guide to MS
Low dose naltrexone
Linoleic acid
Mitoxantrone
MS: What does it mean for me?
Natalizumab (Tysabri)
Pain
Sativex
Sexuality and MS: a guide for women
Spasticity and spasms

Stem cells
Talking about MS
Understanding NICE Guidance

Books

J. Bailey, *Exercise and Physiotherapy*, Multiple Sclerosis Society, London

Cynthia Benz and Richard Reynolds, *Coping with Multiple Sclerosis: a practical guide to understanding and living with MS*. Vermillion, London

Liz Betts, *Exercises for People with MS*, MS Trust, Letchworth

Allen C Bowling, *Complementary and Alternative Medicine and Multiple Sclerosis*, 2nd ed. Demos Medical Publishing, New York

Alistair Compston, Ian McDonald, John Noseworthy et al. *McApline's Multiple Sclerosis*, 4th ed. Churchill Livingstone, Edinburgh

Patricia Coyle and June Halper, *Living with Progressive Multiple Sclerosis: overcoming the challenges*, 2nd ed, Demos Medical Publishing, New York

The Disability Alliance, *Disability Rights Handbook* (updated annually), Disability Alliance, London

Ezard Ernst, Max Pittler and Barbara Wider, *The desktop guide to complementary and alternative medicine: an evidence-based approach – 2nd ed.* Elsevier-Mosby, Edinburgh

Jeffrey Gingold, *Mental Sharpening Stones: managing the cognitive challenges of Multiple Sclerosis*. Demos Medical Publishing, New York

Jeffrey Gingold, *Facing the Cognitive Challenges of Multiple Sclerosis*. Demos Medical Publishing, New York

Rita Greer, *Soft Options for Adults who have Difficulty Chewing*. Souvenir Press, London

Brad Hamler, *Exercises for Multiple Sclerosis*, Healthy Living Books, New York

Gary Hetherington and Carol Young, *My Dad's got MS*. MS Trust, Letchworth

Nancy Holland, Murray Jock and Stephen Reingold, *Multiple Sclerosis: a guide for the newly diagnosed*, 3rd ed. Demos Medical Publishing, New York

Jon Kabat-Zinn, *Full catastrophe living: how to cope with stress, pain and illness using mindfulness meditation*. Piatkus, London

Rosalind Kalb, *Multiple Sclerosis: a guide for families*. Demos Medical Publishing, New York

Gillian Kemp, *Relatively speaking: suggestions to help the long distance carer*. Millwood Books, Hatfield

Rosie Laidlaw, *MS in Your Life: a guide for young carers*. Multiple Sclerosis Society, London

Jane Matthews, *The carer's handbook: essential information and support for all those in a caring role*, 2nd ed. Begbroke 'How to Books', Oxford

Eva McCracken, *Walking on wheels: 50 wheel-friendly trails in Scotland*. Cualann Press, Dunfermline

Motability, *The Rough Guide to Accessible Britain*, Rough Guide Publications, London

Kerry Mutch, *The Young Person's Guide to MS*. MS Trust, Letchworth

M. Pinder, *Complementary Healthcare: a guide for patients*, The Prince of Wales' Foundation, London

Chris Polman, *Multiple Sclerosis: the guide to treatment and management*, 6th edn. Demos Medical Publishing, New York

RADAR, *Holidays in Britain and Ireland: a guide for disabled people*. RADAR, London

Joanna Ridley, Caring for someone with MS: a handbook for family and friends. Multiple Sclerosis Society, London

Penny Sayer and Carolyn Young, *My Mum's got MS*. Roby Education Ltd, Ormskirk

R.T. Shapiro, *Managing the Symptoms of Multiple Sclerosis*, Demos Medical Publishing, New York

Tourism for All, *Easy Access Britain: the guide to accessible places to stay*. Tourism for All, Kendal

Michele Wates, *Disabled Parents: dispelling the myths*. National Childbirth Trust, London

Donna Weihofen, Joanne Robbins and Paula Sullivan, *Easy-to-swallow, Easy-to-chew Cookbook: over 150 tasty and nutritious recipes for people who have difficulty swallowing*. John Wiley, New York

Sally West, *Your Rights to Money Benefits* (regularly updated), Age Concern, London

DVDs

Annie & Dan talk about MS: a DVD for children under 10. Available from the Multiple Sclerosis Society, London

Move it for MS. Exercise DVD featuring Mr Motivator. Available from the MS Trust, Letchworth.

MS Together. The MS Trust's first DVD contains clear and concise information about MS. It features contributions from a range of leading healthcare professionals and interviews with people with MS, sharing personal reflections and experience of living with MS. Available from the MS Trust, Letchworth.

Yoga for MS and Related Conditions. Exercise video for people with limited mobility. Mobility Limited, Canada.

Appendix 3
The Revised McDonald Criteria

The McDonald criteria are named after Professor Ian McDonald the Chairman of the original group of MS experts who published their guidelines for the diagnosis of MS in 2001. These were revised in 2005. They are the latest attempt to distil the essential requirements for a diagnosis of MS and it is important to note that these are consensus guidelines for the diagnosis of MS in adult, Western populations.

Revised McDonald Criteria for diagnosing relapsing-remitting MS

Table A3.1 outlines various scenarios, and shows how MRI scans and other tests can be used to help in reaching a diagnosis of relapsing-remitting MS. You can see that the diagnosis of MS still remains largely clinical, requiring demonstration of the spread or dissemination of lesions of the central nervous system in time and space. If there isn't evidence of at least two clinical attacks and at least two lesions on clinical examination by your neurologist, then MRI and lumbar puncture for cerebrospinal fluid (CSF) can be helpful in providing the additional information required. They are complementary to careful clinical assessment, and are *not* a substitute for it. It must be stressed explicitly that no test or group of tests is 100 per cent specific for MS, and there should be no better explanation for your symptoms and signs.

Positive CSF means either the presence of oligoclonal bands or a raised CSF immunoglobulin index (indicating there is more antibody in the spinal fluid relative to the protein albumin in the spinal fluid than there is in the serum).

Revised McDonald Criteria for diagnosing primary progressive MS

For a diagnosis of primary progressive MS, the 2005 Revised McDonald criteria requires at least one year of progressive neurological deterioration, which can be determined either retrospectively or prospectively from the time a person is first assessed. Then two out of the following three indications are required:

Table A3.1 Simplified Revised 2005 McDonald Criteria for the diagnosis of relapsing-remitting MS

Clinical attacks	Different CNS lesions confirmed on clinical examination	Additional requirements to make MS diagnosis (simplified) [marked by an X]			
		MRI dissemination in Time	MRI dissemination in Space	Positive CSF	OR Requires second clinical attack
2 or more	2 or more	NONE	NONE	NONE	NONE
2 or more	1			X	X
1	2 or more	X			X
1	1	X	X	X	X

Key: CNS = Central nervous system (brain and spinal cord); CSF = Cerebrospinal fluid; Lesion = Area of inflammation

- *Either:*

  A positive brain scan indicating either a GAD enhancing lesion*, or a minimum of nine T2 lesions

  Or:

  A positive brain scan indicating between four and eight T2 lesions**, *and* a positive VER showing a delayed but well-preserved waveform.

- A positive spinal cord MRI indicating two or more T2 lesions

- Positive cerebrospinal fluid (CSF) showing oligoclonal bands or a raised immunoglobulin index.

Notes

** Gadolinium is a substance which is injected into the vein at the time of an MRI scan. It leaks into the brain, 'lighting up' only the areas where the barrier between the blood and the brain (the 'blood-brain barrier') is disrupted, as it can be for a few weeks after an attack of inflammation. Therefore gadolinium can demonstrate newer areas of inflammation which are said to *enhance.*

** T2 lesions refer to areas of inflammation visible on a particular sequence on standard MRI scans that does not require the administration of gadolinium.

| Appendix 4
ABN/NICE treatment guidelines

Guidelines for the use of the beta-interferons and glatiramer acetate
Association of British Neurologists (ABN), January 2001

Beta-interferon (Avonex, Betaferon*, Rebif 22/44)

Starting criteria

Relapsing-remitting MS:

1. Able to walk independently

2. At least two clinically significant relapses in the last two years

Secondary progressive MS:

1. Able to walk at least 10 metres with or without assistance

2. At least two disabling relapses in the last two years

3. Any increase in disability due to slow progression over the last two years has been minimal

The ABN recommends beta-interferon should be offered to patients who fulfil these criteria. It is *not* recommended for patients with clinically isolated syndromes or primary progressive MS.

Stopping criteria

Discontinuation of treatment may become necessary because of intolerable side effects or when a pregnancy is planned. Treatment should also be discontinued when it is no longer effective. The following features are likely to indicate lack of efficacy and should normally be used as stopping criteria:

1. Two disabling relapses, as defined by the examining neurologist, within a 12-month period

2. Secondary progression with an increase in disability observable over 6 months

3. Loss of ability to walk, with or without assistance, persistent for at least 6 months

Glatiramer acetate (Copaxone)

Starting criteria

Relapsing-remitting MS:

1. Able to walk at least 100 metres without assistance

2. At least two clinically significant relapses in the last two years

The ABN recommends glatiramer acetate should be offered to patients who fulfil these criteria. It is *not* recommended for patients with clinically isolated syndromes, secondary progressive MS or primary progressive MS.

Stopping criteria

Discontinuation of treatment may become necessary because of intolerable side effects or when a pregnancy is planned. Treatment should also be discontinued when it is no longer effective. The following features are likely to indicate lack of efficacy and should normally be used as stopping criteria:

1. Two disabling relapses, as defined by the examining neurologist, within a 12-month period

2. Secondary progression with an increase in disability observable over 6 months

3. Loss of ability to walk, with or without assistance, persistent for at least 6 months

Notes

* Also includes Extavia, since 2009.

Beta-interferon and glatiramer acetate are *not* approved by the National Institute for Health and Clinical Excellence (NICE). They are currently available on the NHS for patients who meet 2001 ABN guidelines in accordance with the Department of Health Risk-Sharing Scheme. In March 2007, the Association of British Neurologists issued revised guidelines. At the time of writing, these revised guidelines were withdrawn for immediate review.

Natalizumab for the treatment of adults with highly active relapsing-remitting MS

National Institute for Health and Clinical Excellence (NICE), August 2007

Starting criteria

Natalizumab (Tysabri) is recommended as an option for the treatment only of rapidly evolving severe relapsing-remitting MS. This is defined by two or more disabling relapses in 1 year, and one or more gadolinium-enhancing lesions on brain magnetic resonance imaging (MRI) or a significant increase in T2 lesion load compared with a previous MRI.

Note

At the time of writing, natalizumab is the *only* disease-modifying drug approved by the National Institute for Health and Clinical Excellence (NICE) for use in MS. It is available on the NHS for those patients who meet NICE criteria.

| Index

PRIORITY ORDER FORM

Cut out or photocopy this form and send it (post free in the UK) to:

Class Publishing   **Tel: 01256 302 699**
FREEPOST 16705
Macmillan Distribution   **Fax: 01256 812 558**
Basingstoke RG21 6ZZ

Please send me urgently   *Post included*
(tick below)   *price per copy (UK only)*

☐ **Multiple sclerosis: Answers at your fingertips** (ISBN 978 1 85959 218 2)   £20.99

☐ **Managing your multiple sclerosis** (ISBN 978 1 85959 071 3)   £17.99

☐ **Beating depression** (ISBN 978 1 85959 150 5)   £20.99

☐ **Alzheimer's and other dementias: Answers at your fingertips**   £17.99
(ISBN 978 1 85959 148 2)

☐ **Menopause: Answers at your fingertips** (ISBN 978 1 85959 155 0)   £20.99

☐ **IBS: Answers at your fingertips** (ISBN 978 1 85959 156 7)   £20.99

☐ **Heart health: Answers at your fingertips** (ISBN 978 1 85959 157 4)   £20.99

TOTAL _____

Easy ways to pay

Cheque: I enclose a cheque payable to Class Publishing for £ _____

Credit card: Please debit my   ☐ Mastercard   ☐ Visa   ☐ Amex

Number _____   Expiry date _____

Name _____

My address for delivery is _____

_____

Town _____ County _____ Postcode _____

Telephone number (*in case of query*) _____

Credit card billing address if different from above _____

_____

Town _____ County _____ Postcode _____

Class Publishing's guarantee: remember that if, for any reason, you are not satisfied with these books, we will refund all your money, without any questions asked. Prices and VAT rates may be altered for reasons beyond our control.

The *Class Health* Feedback Form

We hope that you found this ***Class Health*** book helpful. We always appreciate readers' opinions and would be grateful if you could take a few minutes to complete this form for us.

❶ How did you acquire your copy of this book?

From my local library   ☐

Read an article in a newspaper/magazine   ☐

Found it by chance   ☐

Recommended by a friend   ☐

Recommended by a patient organisation/charity   ☐

Recommended by a doctor/nurse/advisor   ☐

Saw an advertisement   ☐

❷ How much of the book have you read?

All of it   ☐

More than half of it   ☐

Less than half of it   ☐

❸ Which chapters have been most helpful?

....

....

❹ Overall, how useful to you was this *Class Health* book?

Extremely useful   ☐

Very useful   ☐

Useful   ☐

❺ What did you find most helpful?

....

....

6 **What did you find least helpful?**

....

....

7 **Have you read any other health books?**

Yes ☐   No ☐

If yes, which subjects did they cover?

....

....

....

How did this *Class Health* book compare?

Much better   ☐

Better   ☐

About the same   ☐

Not as good   ☐

8 **Would you recommend this book to a friend?**

Yes ☐   No ☐

Thank you for your help. Please send your completed form to:

Class Publishing, FREEPOST, London W6 7BR

Surname _____ First name _____

Title Prof/Dr/Mr/Mrs/Ms _____

Address _____

Town _____ Postcode _____ Country _____

☐ Please add my name and address to receive details of related books
[*Please note, we will not pass on your details to any other company*]

Have you found *Multiple sclerosis: Answers at your fingertips* useful and practical? If so, you may be interested in other books from Class Publishing.

**MANAGING YOUR
MULTIPLE SCLEROSIS**   £14.99

*Professor Ian Robinson
and Dr Frank Clifford Rose*

This informative book provides clear and practical advice on many aspects of MS, ranging from dealing with symptoms, to medical management and coping with the issues of everyday living. Topics covered in detail include treatments, employment, finances, home adaptations, pregnancy and childbirth, and complementary therapies.

BEATING DEPRESSION   £17.99

*Dr Stefan Cembrowicz
and Dr Dorcas Kingham*

Depression is one of most common illnesses in the world – affecting up to one in four people at some time in their lives. This book shows sufferers and their families that they are not alone, and offers tried and tested techniques for overcoming depression.

'All you need to know about depression, presented in a clear, concise and readable way.'

ANN DAWSON,
World Health Organization

ALZHEIMER'S AND OTHER DEMENTIAS
Answers at your fingertips   £14.99

*Harry Cayton, Dr Nori Graham
and Dr James Warner*

If you have been affected by dementia, this book is for you. You may have been recently diagnosed, you may know someone who is experiencing symptoms, or you may be caring for someone with the condition.

This book answers over 270 questions about the realities of dementia from people in all these situations. It will help you to understand the condition and take control.

'An invaluable contribution to understanding all forms of dementia.'
Dr JONATHAN MILLER CBE, President
of the Alzheimer's Disease Society

MENOPAUSE
Answers at your fingertips   £17.99

Dr Heather Currie

The average age of the menopause is 51 years, but it can occur much earlier or later. The symptoms vary widely in their severity, and can include hot flushes, night sweats, palpitations, insomnia, joint pain and headaches. Women are at greater risk of osteoporosis after the menopause.

This invaluable guide answers hundreds of questions from women and provides positive, practical advice on a range of issues.

IBS
Answers at your fingertips   £17.99

Dr Ehoud Shmueli

Irritable bowel syndrome (IBS) is often dismissed as a trivial complaint, but the reality is very different. IBS is an extremely common and distressing condition affecting up to 20% of us at any one time.

If you have IBS, this book will answer the questions you may have been too embarrassed to ask. It provides detailed advice on all aspects of the condition, answering over 430 questions from people with IBS.

HEART HEALTH
Answers at your fingertips   £17

Dr Graham Jackson

This practical handbook, written by a leading cardiologist, answers all your questions about heart conditions. It tell you all about you and your heart; how keep your heart healthy, or if it has be affected by heart disease, how to ma as strong as possible.

'Those readers who want to know about the various treatments for disease will be much enlightene
Dr JAN
The Do